Workbook for

# Pilbeam's Mechanical Ventilation

## Physiological and Clinical Applications

*Eighth Edition*

Workbook for

# Pilbeam's Mechanical Ventilation

## Physiological and Clinical Applications

*Eighth Edition*

**J.M. Cairo, PhD, RRT, FAARC**
Dean Emeritus and Professor
Louisiana State University Health Sciences Center
New Orleans, Louisiana

**Sandra T. Hinski, PhD, RRT-NPS**
Dean, Career and Technical Education
Academic Affairs
Paradise Valley Community College
Phoenix, Arizona

ELSEVIER

Elsevier
3251 Riverport Lane
St. Louis, Missouri 63043

WORKBOOK FOR PILBEAM'S MECHANICAL VENTILATION:
PHYSIOLOGICAL AND CLINICAL APPLICATIONS, EIGHTH EDITION          ISBN: 978-0-323-87169-3

---

**Notice**

---

Previous editions copyrighted 2020, 2016, 2012, 2006 and 1999.

*Content Strategist:* Melissa Rawe
*Senior Content Development Manager:* Laura Schmidt
*Content Development Specialist:* Kristen Helm
*Publishing Services Manager:* Deepthi Unni
*Project Manager:* Thoufiq Mohammed
*Cover Designer:* Gopalakrishnan Venkataraman

Printed in India

Last digit is the print number: 9  8  7  6  5  4  3  2  1

*To my husband, Bill, and my children, Charlie and Stella, for their tolerance of the long days and nights I spent in my office writing. I love you and thank you. And to all my students for unknowingly pushing me to never stop learning.*

*Sandra T. Hinski*

# Preface

The goal of this workbook is to assist respiratory care students in the mastery of the information presented in *Pilbeam's Mechanical Ventilation: Physiological and Clinical Applications,* Eigth Edition, by James M. Cairo.

Reading any medical textbook requires active participation, which is very different from the passive reading we do for pleasure. The reader should expect to read the material slowly and carefully to aid in the comprehension of the material. You should focus your attention on the information being presented. Reading with a purpose increases concentration, comprehension, retention, and interest in the subject matter.

I recommend that the student use the text and workbook in the following manner:

First, preview or scan through the text by reading the title, outline, objectives, and key terms. Remember: the learning objectives indicate what the author intends for the reader to know after finishing with the chapter. Skim the headings and subheadings. Read the Chapter Summary. This highlights the structure of the chapter and emphasizes important concepts.

Next, turn the title into a question. The idea here is that asking a question focuses your reading on finding information that will help you answer the question. It makes reading a more active search for meaning. Use the review questions in the workbook to help you focus on important points in the chapter. Read carefully (in manageable chunks) to answer these questions. Note important details and relationships of ideas. The review questions in this workbook are based on the author's learning objectives for each chapter. Pay particular attention to the figures, boxes, tables, key points, case studies, and clinical scenarios because they are included to help learn the material.

Then review the textbook's Chapter Review Questions. Be able to answer all of the questions. This will ensure that highlighting or annotating the textbook is being done efficiently.

After this, answer the Critical Thinking Questions and the Case Study Questions in the Workbook. This will help with analysis and application-type questions seen on the board exams. Re-read any topic you are struggling with to ensure your understanding of the concept. The next step is to attempt the NBRC-Style Questions. Once you have read a chapter or topic, try reading peer-reviewed literature on the subject that includes experiments and case studies. This will help you apply your reading into the real world of respiratory care. And never forget to ask for help sooner rather than later if a topic is just not sinking in. ***All answers for the workbook are available through your instructor via the Evolve website.***

**Sandra T. Hinski, M.S., RRT-NPS**

# Contents

# 1 Basic Terms and Concepts of Mechanical Ventilation

## LEARNING OBJECTIVES

*On completion of this chapter the reader will be able to do the following:*

1. Define *ventilation, external respiration,* and *internal respiration.*
2. Draw a graph showing how intrapleural and alveolar (intrapulmonary) pressures change during spontaneous ventilation and during a positive pressure breath.
3. Define the terms *transpulmonary pressure, transrespiratory pressure, transairway pressure, transthoracic pressure, elastance, compliance,* and *resistance.*
4. Provide the value for intraalveolar pressure throughout inspiration and expiration during normal, quiet breathing.
5. Write the formulas for calculating compliance and resistance.
6. Explain how changes in lung compliance affect the peak pressure measured during inspiration with a mechanical ventilator.
7. Describe the changes in airway conditions that can lead to increased resistance.
8. Calculate the airway resistance given the peak inspiratory pressure, a plateau pressure, and the flow rate.
9. Using a figure showing abnormal compliance or airway resistance, determine which lung unit will fill more quickly or with a greater volume.
10. Compare several time constants, and explain how different time constants will affect volume distribution during inspiration.
11. Give the percentage of passive filling (or emptying) for one, two, three, and five time- constants.
12. Briefly discuss the principle of operation of negative pressure, positive pressure, and high-frequency mechanical ventilators.
13. Define peak inspiratory pressure, baseline pressure, positive end-expiratory pressure, and plateau pressure.
14. Describe the measurement of plateau pressure.

**KEY TERMS CROSSWORD PUZZLE**

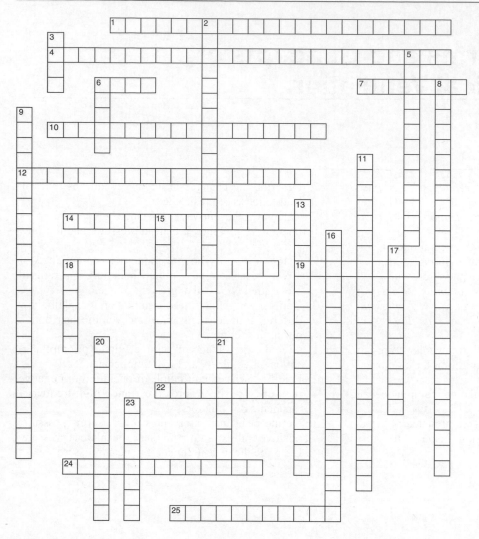

**Down**

2 Pressure measured at the mouth (three words)
3 Abbreviation for ventilation using small pulses of pressurized gas at rates between 100 and 400 breaths/min
5 Complication of positive pressure ventilation that causes an inadvertent buildup of positive pressure in the alveoli (two words)
6 Abbreviation for ventilation using lower-than-normal tidal volumes and respiratory rates between 60 and 100 breaths/min

**Across**

1 Alternate term for pressure in the airways of the lungs (three words)
4 Total amount of gas remaining in the lungs after a resting expiration (three words)
6 Abbreviation for a form of ventilatory support characterized by rates of up to 4000 breaths/min
7 Pressure measurement when there is no gas flow
10 Pressure measured in the esophagus that is used to represent intrapleural pressure (two words)
12 Movement of oxygen into cells and of carbon dioxide out of cells (two words)
14 Measurement of elastic forces that oppose lung inflation (two words)
18 Pressure in the airways of the lungs (two words)
19 Another term for intrinsic PEEP (hyphenated word)
22 Impedance of gas flow through the conductive airways
24 Deliberate increase in the ventilator's baseline pressure (two words)
25 Movement of gas molecules across a membrane

8 Pressure between the alveolus and the pleural space responsible for maintaining alveolar inflation (three words)
9 Another term for the highest pressure recorded at the end of inspiration (three words)
11 Airway communications between the lung and the pleural space (two words)
13 Highest pressure recorded at the end of inspiration (three words)
15 The ease with which the lungs distend
16 Movement of oxygen into the bloodstream and carbon dioxide out of the bloodstream (two words)
17 Movement of air into the lungs for gas exchange and out of the lungs for carbon dioxide removal
18 Functional unit of the lung
20 Mathematical expression used to describe the filling and emptying of lung units (two words)
21 Tendency of the lungs to return to their original form after being stretched
23 Difference between an area of high pressure and low pressure

## CHAPTER REVIEW QUESTIONS

1. Describe the difference between ventilation and respiration.

   _____

   _____

   _____

   _____

2. The diffusion of oxygen and carbon dioxide in and out of the alveolar capillaries is known as _____, whereas the exchange of oxygen and carbon dioxide between the systemic capillaries and the cells of the body is called _____.

3. Describe what happens during quiet expiration.

4. The pressure in the potential space between the parietal and visceral pleura is known as _____. At the end of exhalation during spontaneous breathing, this pressure is approximately _____, and at the end of inspiration, it is about _____.

5. Use Figure 1.1 in your text book for this question.

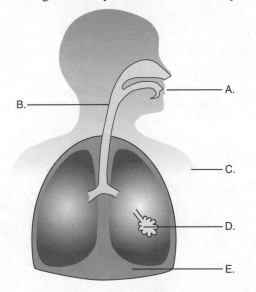

   a. Identify the pressures labeled *A* through *E*.

   _____

   b. Name at least three additional terms for pressure *A*.

   1. _____

   2. _____

   3. _____

6. How is intrapleural pressure (Ppl) estimated?

   _____

   _____

7. The pressure gradient between the airway opening and the alveolus is known as _____. This pressure is responsible for the movement of air in the _____. This gradient is calculated by the formula _____ _____.

8. The pressure required to expand or contract the lungs and the chest wall at the same time is _____. This pressure gradient is calculated by the formula _____.

9. The pressure required to maintain alveolar inflation is known as _____ and is calculated by the formula _____.

10. The pressure that is required for inflation of the lungs during positive pressure ventilation is called _____ and is calculated by the formula _____.

11. Use Figure 1.1 to answer questions a through d.

    a. What pressure gradient is represented by Point A to Point C? What is its function during breathing?

    _____

    _____

    b. What pressure gradient is represented by Point C to Point D? What is its function during breathing?

    _____

    _____

    c. What pressure gradient is represented by Point D to Point E? What is its function during breathing?

    _____

    _____

    d. What pressure gradient is represented by Point B to Point D? What is its function during breathing?

    _____

    _____

12. On the graph in Figure 1.2, label the *x*- and *y*-axes, draw the changes in $P_{alv}$ during a spontaneous breath, and label inspiration and expiration.

13. Describe how a negative pressure ventilator causes air to move into an individual's lungs.

    _____

    _____

    _____

    _____

14. List three advantages of using negative pressure ventilators.

    1. _____

    2. _____

    3. _____

15. Calculate the transairway pressure ($P_{TA}$) when the mouth pressure ($P_M$) is $+25$ cm $H_2O$ and the $P_{alv}$ is $+5$ cm $H_2O$.

    _____

16. Draw and label, on the graph in Figure 1.3, the changes in intrapulmonary pressure that occur during a positive pressure breath with a PIP of 30 cm $H_2O$, a $P_{plat}$ of 20 cm $H_2O$, a PEEP of 5 cm $H_2O$, inspiratory time of 2 seconds, and expiratory time of 4 seconds.

17. Draw and label, on the graph in Figure 1.4, the changes in intrapulmonary pressure that occur during a positive pressure breath with a PIP of 45 cm $H_2O$, a $P_{plat}$ of 25 cm $H_2O$, a PEEP of 10 cm $H_2O$, inspiratory time of 1 second, and expiratory time of 2 seconds, followed by a spontaneous breath with the same baseline.

18. The highest pressure recorded at the end of inspiration is called _____ or _____.

19. The pressure at which expiration ends is called _____.

20. When the end expiratory pressure is above the atmospheric pressure, it is called _____.

21. The pressure required to overcome the elastic recoil of the lungs is known as _____ and is measured on a mechanically ventilated person by _____.

22. What are the two types of forces that oppose inflation of the lungs?

23. The relative ease with which a structure distends is known as _____, and the tendency of a structure to return to its original form after being stretched is known as _____.

24. Pulmonary compliance is defined as _____, and the formula is written as _____.

25. Normally, the total compliance of the lungs and the thorax is about _____, but it can range from _____ to _____.

26. While mechanically ventilated, the compliance value for a male with normal lungs is _____, and for a female with normal lungs is _____.

27. What is the formula used to calculate static compliance?

    _____

28. When more pressure is required to deliver a set tidal volume ($V_T$), what is likely happening to compliance?

    _____

29. Calculate the static compliance when $P_{plat}$ is 27 cm $H_2O$, baseline pressure is 10 cm $H_2O$, and $V_T$ is 750 mL.

    _____

30. Calculate the static compliance when $P_{plat}$ is 35 cm $H_2O$, baseline pressure is 5 cm $H_2O$, and $V_T$ is 575 mL.

    _____

31. Calculate the static compliance when $P_{plat}$ is 18 cm $H_2O$, baseline pressure is 0 cm $H_2O$, and $V_T$ is 650 mL.

    _____

32. What happens to PIP as the lungs become more difficult to ventilate? What happens to the lung compliance?

    _____

33. Define *resistance*.

    _____

34. What is the formula for airway resistance ($R_{aw}$)?

    _____

35. What is the normal resistance range for flow rates of 0.5 L/s?

    _____

36. What lung disease causes both airway resistance and static compliance to increase?

    _____

37. Calculate the $P_{TA}$ when PIP is 27 cm $H_2O$ and $P_{plat}$ is 20 cm $H_2O$.

    _____

38. How much pressure is needed to overcome airway resistance when PIP is 30 cm $H_2O$ and $P_{plat}$ is 20 cm $H_2O$?

_____

39. What is the normal amount of pressure lost to airway resistance when a patient has a properly sized endotracheal tube?

_____

40. Calculate $R_{aw}$ for a ventilated patient with the following: PIP 48 cm $H_2O$, $P_{plat}$ 30 cm $H_2O$, and a set flow rate of 40 L/min.

_____

_____

41. Calculate airway resistance for a ventilated patient with the following: PIP 25 cm $H_2O$, $P_{plat}$ 15 cm $H_2O$, and a set flow rate of 60 L/min.

_____

42. Why are the characteristics of the lung not homogenous?

_____

_____

43. Compare the filling time and volume for a normal lung unit, a low compliance unit, and a unit with a high airway resistance using the same driving pressure.

_____

_____

_____

_____

44. What factors contribute to resistance when breathing?

_____

_____

45. What clinical factors can increase the airway resistance by decreasing the radius of the airways?

_____

_____

46. How many seconds will it take to allow 86% of the $V_T$ to be exhaled when the compliance is 25 mL/cm $H_2O$ and the resistance is 30 cm $H_2O$/L/s?

_____

_____

47. Calculate the time constant for a mechanically ventilated patient when $V_T$ is 600 mL, PIP is 30 cm $H_2O$, $P_{plat}$ is 24 cm $H_2O$, and flow rate is 60 L/min, with no PEEP.

_____

_____

_____

_____

48. What percentage of passive filling occurs for 1, 2, 3, 4, and 5 time constants?

_____

_____

49. The time constant for patient #1 is 0.05 second; patient #2 is 3 seconds; and 0.5 second for patient #3. If the same filling pressure is used for each, which patient will receive the most volume during inspiration and why?

_____

_____

_____

50. Calculate the time constant for a compliance of 55 mL/cm $H_2O$ and a resistance of 6 cm $H_2O$/L/s.

_____

_____

51. What is the inspiratory time setting to allow 95% volume emptying for a patient with the time constant calculated in Question 50?

_____

52. Why can patients with increased airway resistance develop air trapping when ventilator rates are set too high?

_____

_____

53. Calculate the time constant for a mechanically ventilated patient when the $V_T$ is 700 mL, PIP is 45 cm $H_2O$, $P_{plat}$ is 18 cm $H_2O$, flow rate is 60 L/min, and PEEP is 5 cm $H_2O$.

_____

_____

_____

_____

54. Which of the two lung units represented in Figure 1.5 will receive more volume, given the same amount of time for inspiration? Explain your answer.

A          B

_____

_____

_____

_____

55. Which of the two lung units represented in Figure 1.6 will fill more quickly? Explain your answer.

_____

_____

_____

_____

**CRITICAL THINKING QUESTIONS**

1. When the PIP is 43 cm $H_2O$ and the $P_{plat}$ is 18 cm $H_2O$, how much pressure is required to overcome the resistance of the airways?

_____

_____

_____

2. What time constants would you expect for a patient with adult respiratory distress syndrome?

_____

_____

_____

3. Describe how emphysema causes lung units to have long time constants.

_____

_____

_____

4. What time constants would you expect for a 30-week (gestational age) premature infant?

_____

5. When measuring the $P_{plat}$ on a patient receiving mechanical ventilation, you observe a $P_{plat}$ that is higher than the PIP. What is one explanation for this?

_____

_____

_____

_____

## CASE STUDIES

### Case Study 1

A respiratory therapist reviews the following information concerning an intubated patient being mechanically ventilated.

| Time | PIP | $P_{plat}$ | $V_T$ | Set Flow Rate | PEEP |
|------|-----|-----------|-------|---------------|------|
| 0800 | 18 cm $H_2O$ | 10 cm $H_2O$ | 600 mL | 45 L/min | 5 cm $H_2O$ |
| 1000 | 24 cm $H_2O$ | 12 cm $H_2O$ | 600 mL | 45 L/min | 5 cm $H_2O$ |
| 1200 | 35 cm $H_2O$ | 11 cm $H_2O$ | 600 mL | 45 L/min | 5 cm $H_2O$ |

1. What is the $P_{TA}$ at 0800, 1000, and 1200?

_____

_____

2. Calculate the $R_{aw}$ at 0800, 1200, and 1200.

_____

_____

_____

_____

_____

3. Calculate the static compliance at 0800, 1000, and 1200.

_____

_____

_____

_____

_____

4. Calculate one time constant at 0800, 1000, and 1200.

_____

_____

_____

5. a. What caused the PIP to rise between 0800 and 1200?

_____

  b. What problems will this cause when ventilating the patient?

_____

_____

_____

_____

### Case Study 2

The following information is obtained from the flow sheet of an intubated patient being mechanically ventilated.

| Time | PIP | $P_{plat}$ | $V_T$ | Set Flow Rate | PEEP |
|------|-----|-----------|-------|---------------|------|
| 1000 | 40 cm $H_2O$ | 28 cm $H_2O$ | 550 mL | 40 L/min | 0 cm $H_2O$ |
| 1200 | 47 cm $H_2O$ | 37 cm $H_2O$ | 550 mL | 40 L/min | 5 cm $H_2O$ |
| 1400 | 54 cm $H_2O$ | 43 cm $H_2O$ | 550 mL | 40 L/min | 7 cm $H_2O$ |
| 1600 | 45 cm $H_2O$ | 33 cm $H_2O$ | 450 mL | 60 L/min | 12 cm $H_2O$ |

1. Complete the table below.

| Time | $P_{TA}$ | $R_{aw}$ | $C_{STAT}$ | Time Constant |
|------|----------|----------|------------|---------------|
| 1000 | | | | |
| 1200 | | | | |
| 1400 | | | | |
| 1600 | | | | |

2. What is the source of the rising PIP between 1000 and 1400?

_____

_____

3. What would be the minimum inspiratory time for this patient at 1600 hours?

_____

_____

## NBRC-STYLE QUESTIONS

1. Calculate the static effective compliance during the delivery of a ventilator breath with 650 mL with a $P_{plat}$ of 28 cm $H_2O$ and a PEEP of 0.
   a. 0.04 cm $H_2O$/L
   b. 0.23 L/cm $H_2O$
   c. mL/cm $H_2O$
   d. Not enough information is given

2. Calculate the $R_{aw}$ for a patient receiving mechanical ventilation with a set $V_T$ of 825 mL and a peak flow setting of 50 L/min when the PIP is 46 cm $H_2O$ and the $P_{plat}$ is 22 cm $H_2O$.
   a. 13.7 cm $H_2O$/L/s
   b. 26.5 cm $H_2O$/L/s
   c. 28.9 cm $H_2O$/L/s
   d. 38.2 cm $H_2O$/L/s

3. Calculate one time constant for the following data:
   PIP: 29 cm $H_2O$
   $P_{plat}$: 23 cm $H_2O$
   $V_T$: 600 cc
   PEEP: 5 cm $H_2O$
   Inspiratory flow rate: 45 L/min
   a. 0.017 second
   b. 0.021 second
   c. 0.21 second
   d. 0.27 second

4. The cause of a mechanically ventilated patient's PIP increasing from 20 to 40 cm $H_2O$ while the static compliance remains relatively unchanged is which of the following?
   a. Removed mucous plugs
   b. Increased $R_{aw}$
   c. Tension pneumothorax
   d. Decreased elastance

5. An increase in PIP and $P_{plat}$ with a stable $P_{TA}$ may be caused by which of the following?
   a. Acute respiratory distress syndrome
   b. Acute asthma exacerbation
   c. Retained secretions in the airways
   d. An endotracheal tube that is too small

6. Which of the following will occur when a patient's lung-thoracic compliance improves?
   1. $P_{plat}$ decreases
   2. PIP decreases
   3. $P_{plat}$ increases
   4. $P_{TA}$ increases
   a. 1 and 2 only
   b. 1 and 4 only
   c. 2 and 3 only
   d. 3 and 4 only

7. Over the course of several hours, a respiratory therapist has detected an increase in the $P_{TA}$ of a mechanically ventilated patient. The patient's $P_{plat}$ has remained stable. Which of the following may be the cause of this increase?
   a. Improving lung-thoracic compliance
   b. Acute respiratory distress syndrome
   c. Fluid buildup in the peritoneal cavity
   d. Increase of airway secretions

8. A patient's $P_{TA}$ is rising while the $P_{plat}$ is constant. Which of the following should be done to correct this problem?
   1. Administer a bronchodilator.
   2. Place a large-bore needle in the third intercostals space.
   3. Measure the auto-PEEP.
   4. Suction airway secretions.
   a. 2 only
   b. 3 and 4 only
   c. 1 and 4 only
   d. 1 and 3 only

9. Calculate the static compliance for a patient who is being mechanically ventilated and has an exhaled $V_T$ of 825 mL, a $P_{plat}$ of 47 cm $H_2O$, and a PEEP of 8 cm $H_2O$.
   a. 15 mL/cm $H_2O$
   b. 18 mL/cm $H_2O$
   c. 21 mL/cm $H_2O$
   d. 47 mL/cm $H_2O$

10. Which of the following situations will demonstrate the highest airway resistance?
   a. PIP is 65 cm $H_2O$, $P_{plat}$ is 55 cm $H_2O$, flow rate is 60 L/min
   b. PIP is 52 cm $H_2O$, $P_{plat}$ is 18 cm $H_2O$, flow rate is 45 L/min
   c. PIP is 45 cm $H_2O$, $P_{plat}$ is 30 cm $H_2O$, flow rate is 50 L/min
   d. PIP is 30 cm $H_2O$, $P_{plat}$ is 10 cm $H_2O$, flow rate is 40 L/min

# 2 How Ventilators Work

## LEARNING OBJECTIVES

*On completion of this chapter the reader will be able to do the following:*

1. List the basic types of power sources used for mechanical ventilators.
2. Give examples of ventilators that use an electrical and a pneumatic power source.
3. Explain the difference in function between positive and negative pressure ventilators.
4. Distinguish between a closed-loop and an open-loop system.
5. Define *user interface.*
6. Describe a ventilator's internal and external pneumatic circuits.
7. Discuss the difference between a single-circuit and a double-circuit ventilator.
8. Identify the components of an external circuit (patient circuit).
9. Explain the function of an externally mounted exhalation valve.
10. Compare the functions of the three types of volume displacement drive mechanisms.
11. Describe the function of the proportional solenoid valve.

## KEY TERMS PUZZLE

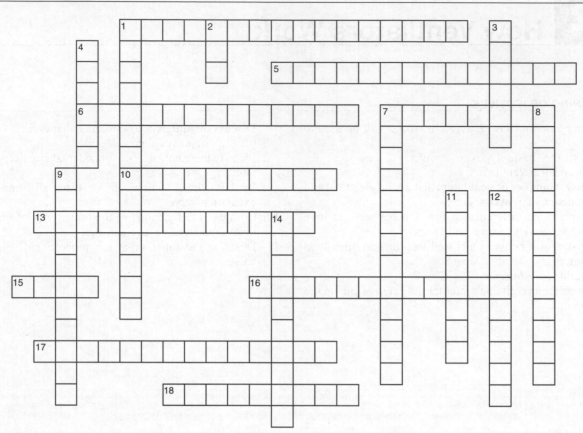

### Across

1 A pathway of tubes within the ventilator is an internal _____ (two words)
5 Single chip made of integrated circuits
6 Another name for the control panel (two words)
7 Pneumatic valve that uses an electromagnetic field and is controlled by a microprocessor
10 Device for which the internal volume can be changed
13 What is inside the black box?
15 Type of controller
16 Stepper motor that controls a hinged clamp device (two words)
17 Mechanical device that causes gas to flow to the patient (two words)
18 Uses 50 psi as a power source

### Down

1 Connects to the patient (two words)
2 Ventilator mode where the clinician sets a minimum minute ventilation (abbreviation)
3 Mechanism to change the internal volume
4 Type of controller
7 From ventilator directly to patient type ventilator (two words)
8 This type of ventilator has two internal pneumatic circuits (two words)
9 Type of valve that controls the gas flow (two words)
11 Unintelligent system (two words)
12 Intelligent system (two words)
13 Uses AC or DC as a power source

## CHAPTER REVIEW QUESTIONS

1. Name the two types of power sources used by ventilators that provide energy to perform the work of ventilating the patient.
   a. _____
   b. _____

2. Which specific power source does each of the following ventilators use?

   Bird Mark 7 _____

   LTV 1150 _____

   LTV 1200 _____

3. Describe an open-loop system.
   _____
   _____

4. Describe a closed-loop system.
   _____
   _____

5. Explain the difference in how gas flows into the lung with positive- versus negative-pressure ventilators.
   _____
   _____
   _____
   _____

6. The position on the ventilator where the clinician inputs and monitors ventilator parameters is known as the _____.

7. List five common components that can be set by the clinician using dials or touch panels located on the user interface of the ventilator.
   a. _____
   b. _____
   c. _____
   d. _____
   e. _____

8. From your answer to Question 7, what four ventilator variables do these controls ultimately regulate?
   a. _____
   b. _____
   c. _____
   d. _____

9. Inside a ventilator, gas flow passes through what type of circuit?
   _____

10. After exiting the ventilator, gas flow passes through the _____ on its way to the patient.

11. The gas flow from the ventilator's power source goes directly to the patient. This is known as what type of internal pneumatic circuit?
    _____

12. Describe the difference between single- and double-circuit ventilators. Which is more common in Intensive Care Unit (ICU) ventilators today?
    _____

13. List the four basic elements of a patient circuit.
    a. _____
    b. _____
    c. _____
    d. _____

14. Identify the labeled parts of the ventilator circuit shown in Figure 2.1.

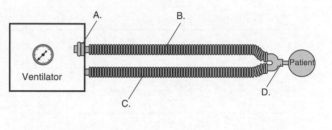

    a. _____
    b. _____
    c. _____
    d. _____

15. Explain how an external exhalation valve operates.
    _____
    _____
    _____
    _____

16. In most current ICU ventilators, where are most exhalation valves located?
    _____

17. What is the drive mechanism?
    _____

18. List two types of flow-control valves available on current ventilators.
    a. _____
    b. _____

19. Describe how each of the flow-control valves operates.
    _____
    _____
    _____
    _____
    _____

20. The internal hardware that converts electrical or pneumatic energy to a system that provides a breath to a patient is called the _____.

21. Name four types of compressors that are used in ventilators.
    a. _____
    b. _____
    c. _____
    d. _____

22. Describe how a spring-loaded bellows functions.
    _____
    _____
    _____

23. Describe how a linear drive piston functions.
    _____
    _____

24. Describe how a rotary drive piston functions.
    _____
    _____
    _____
    _____

25. The ICU ventilators used today have what type of internal functions?
    _____
    _____

## CRITICAL THINKING QUESTIONS

1. If the exhalation valve fails to close, what happens to the inspiratory gas flow?
   _____
   _____

2. What type of ventilator could be used during a magnetic resonance imaging procedure?
   _____
   _____

## CASE STUDIES

### Case Study 1

A patient receiving mechanical ventilation needs to be transported to another medical center for treatment. What type of power source would be appropriate for use during patient transport?

_____

While being mechanically ventilated in a mode that allows spontaneous breathing, a patient becomes apneic. The ventilator automatically alarms and switches to full ventilatory support. Is this an open- or closed-loop system? Explain.

_____
_____
_____

## NBRC-STYLE QUESTIONS

1. The power used by a mechanical ventilator to perform the work of ventilating the patient is known as which of the following?
   a. Force
   b. Pressure
   c. Input power
   d. Output power

2. Which of the following statement(s) is (are) true concerning combined power ventilators?
   1. They must have an electrical power source and two 50-psi gas sources.
   2. They often have RAM and ROM for data and preprogrammed modes.
   3. The electrical power provides the energy to deliver the breath.
   4. The pneumatic power controls the internal function of the machine.
   a. 2 only
   b. 1 and 3 only
   c. 3 and 4 only
   d. 1, 2, and 4 only

3. The internal circuit of a ventilator has the gas go directly from its power source to the patient. This is known as which of the following?
   a. External circuit
   b. Internal circuit
   c. Single circuit
   d. Double circuit

4. One of the functions of the exhalation valve is to do which of the following?
   a. Regulate pressure
   b. Ensure adequate humidification
   c. Ensure gas delivery on inspiration
   d. Determine the patient's tidal volume

5. A closed-loop system is used to guarantee a minute ventilation to a patient. The minute ventilation delivered to the patient differs significantly from the set volume. The ventilator will do which of the following?
   a. Alarm and shut off
   b. Switch to 100% oxygen
   c. Deliver the set minute ventilation
   d. Alter the delivered volume

6. The mechanical device that causes gas to flow to the patient is known as which of the following?
   a. Drive mechanism
   b. Power transmission
   c. Exhalation valve
   d. Solenoid valve

7. Volume displacement devices include which of the following?
   1. Pistons
   2. Stepper motors
   3. Concertina bags
   4. Proportional solenoids
   a. 1 and 4 only
   b. 1 and 3 only
   c. 2 and 3 only
   d. 2 and 4 only

8. The flow-control valve that uses an electromagnetic field is which of the following?
   a. Digital valve
   b. Stepper motor
   c. Solenoid valve
   d. Rotating blade

9. Currently, which type of ventilator is most commonly used in ICU?
   a. Fluidic ventilator
   b. Electrically powered ventilator
   c. Pneumatically powered ventilator
   d. Microprocessor controlled ventilator

10. The volume displacement device that creates a sinusoidal flow wave pattern during inspiration is which of the following?
    a. Spring-loaded bellows
    b. Linear drive piston
    c. Rotary drive piston
    d. Concertina bag

# 3  How a Breath Is Delivered

*On completion of this chapter, the reader will be able to do the following:*

1. Write the equation of motion and define each term in the equation.
2. Give two other names for pressure ventilation and volume ventilation.
3. Compare pressure, volume, and flow delivery in volume-controlled breaths and pressure-controlled breaths.
4. Name the two most commonly used patient-trigger variables.
5. Identify the patient-trigger variable that requires the least work of breathing for a patient receiving mechanical ventilation.
6. Explain the effect on the volume delivered and the inspiratory time if a ventilator reaches the set maximum pressure limit during volume ventilation.
7. Recognize the effects of a critical ventilator circuit leak on pressure readings and volume measurements.
8. Define the effects of inflation hold on inspiratory time.
9. Give an example of a current ventilator that provides negative pressure during part of the expiratory phase.
10. Based on the description of a pressure–time curve, identify a clinical situation in which expiratory resistance is increased.
11. Describe two methods of applying continuous pressure to the airways that can be used to improve oxygenation in patients with refractory hypoxemia.

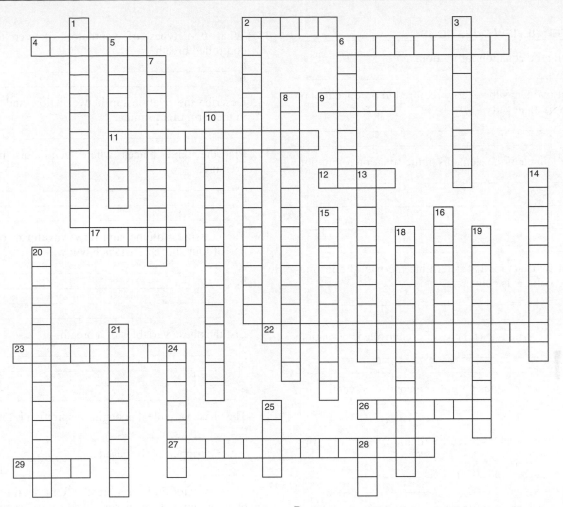

**Across**

2 Variable that ends inspiration
4 Specific amount that begins inspiration
6 Gas law that governs tubing compressibility (two words)
9 Applying positive pressure during expiration during mechanical ventilation (abbreviation)
11 The ventilator begins inspiration (two words)
12 Applying negative pressure during expiration (abbreviation)
17 Maximum value a variable can attain
22 Primary variable the ventilator uses to cause inspiration (two words)
23 Gas speed reaches a maximum amount (two words)
26 Pressure read during an inspiratory pause
27 Maneuver performed to measure auto-PEEP (two words)
29 A baseline pressure at zero (abbreviation)

**Down**

1 Gas speed begins inspiration (two words)
2 The way a ventilator marks the end of inspiration (two words)
3 Most common mechanism for ending inspiration in the pressure support mode (two words)
5 A breath initiated by the ventilator is a _____ breath.
6 Pressure level from which a ventilator breath begins
7 Maxed out at an amount (two words)
8 Pressure target ventilator mode where the patient breathes spontaneously (two words)
10 Ventilator mode where the set limit is pressure (two words)
13 Breathing out
14 The patient is making no effort—ventilation is being _____ by the ventilator.
15 Breathing in
16 Variable that begins inspiration
18 Variable controlling a certain phase of a breath (two words)
19 A breath controlled by the patient
20 A breath begun by the operator (two words)
21 The ventilator ends inspiration (two words)
24 Variable that begins inspiration
25 Application of pressures above ambient throughout inspiration and expiration to a spontaneously breathing patient (abbreviation)
28 Type of ventilation that assists both inspiration and expiration (abbreviation)

**CHAPTER REVIEW QUESTIONS**

1. Write the equation for motion.
   _____

2. List two ways the energy required to produce motion can be achieved.
   a. _____
   b. _____

3. Explain all of the elements of the equation for motion.
   _____
   _____
   _____
   _____

4. List two factors that determine the way the inspiratory volume is delivered.
   a. _____
   b. _____

5. List two synonyms for pressure-controlled ventilation.
   a. _____
   b. _____

6. List two synonyms for volume-controlled ventilation.
   a. _____
   b. _____

7. List four variables that a ventilator can control during inspiration.
   a. _____
   b. _____
   c. _____
   d. _____

8. The primary variable that a ventilator adjusts to produce inspiration is called _____.

9. During pressure-controlled breaths, the compliance and resistance of a patient's lungs change. What happens to volume and flow?
   _____
   _____

10. If during volume-controlled breaths the patient's lung compliance decreases, what will happen to the peak inspiratory pressure (PIP)?
    _____
    _____

11. Explain your answer to Question 10.
    _____
    _____

12. Both pressure and volume waveforms can be affected by changes in lung characteristics while what type of control variable is being used?
    _____

13. What two types of ventilators deliver a time-controlled breath?
    a. _____
    b. _____

14. Describe the relationship between flow and volume in the form of a formula.
    _____

15. List the three places where ventilators measure pressure.
    a. _____
    b. _____
    c. _____

16. The pressure, volume, and flow waveforms can take one of four shapes. List each below.
    a. _____
    b. _____
    c. _____
    d. _____

17. List the phase variables of a breath.
    a. _____
    b. _____
    c. _____
    d. _____

18. The phase variable that begins inspiration is known as the _____.

19. Patient triggering is based on _____, _____, or _____ changes.

20. The ventilator initiates a breath after a set time. What phase variable is this describing?
    _____

21. Describe the limit variable.
    _____

22. Describe the cycle variable. _____

23. Describe the baseline variable. _____

24. Explain auto-triggering.
    _____
    _____

25. At which pressure would it be easier for a patient to initiate a breath? −1 cm $H_2O$ or −3 cm $H_2O$. At which flow would it be easier for a patient to initiate a breath? 2 L/min or 4 L/min. (Circle the correct answers.)

26. If the flow sensitivity is set at 2 L/min and the baseline flow is 6 L/min, at what flow will the ventilator be triggered to give a breath? _____

27. When set properly by the clinician, which triggering method has been shown to require less work of breathing for the patient? _____

28. Describe volume triggering.

_____

_____

Questions 29 through 32 refer to Figure 3.1.

Time (seconds)

29. What is the control variable? _____

30. What is the expiratory time? _____

31. What is the inspiratory time? _____

32. What is the baseline? _____

Questions 33 through 36 refer to Figure 3.2.

Time (seconds)

33. What type of trigger does wave *A* have?

_____

34. What type of trigger does wave *B* have?

_____

35. What type of trigger does wave *C* have?

_____

36. What is the baseline? _____

37. The maximum value that a variable can attain is known as a _____.

Questions 38 through 42: Classify the following breaths as mandatory, assisted, or spontaneous.

38. Pressure-triggered, pressure-limited, time-cycled:

_____

39. Flow-triggered, volume-limited, time-cycled:

_____

40. Time-triggered, pressure-limited, time-cycled:

_____

41. Flow-triggered, patient-cycled:

_____

42. Pressure-triggered, flow-limited, volume-limited, volume-cycled:

_____

43. Do limits cycle a breath? _____

44. When the set high-pressure limit is reached during inspiration, what happens (if using the Covidien PB 840)?

_____

_____

45. List three names ventilator manufacturers use for the maximum pressure-control function.
    a. _____
    b. _____
    c. _____

46. Typically, how does the clinician determine the maximum safety pressure?

_____

47. What is the internal maximum safety pressure used by most ventilator manufacturers?

_____

48. How do most Intensive Care Unit (ICU) ventilators achieve volume cycling?

_____

_____

49. What is the tubing compressibility factor for most adult ventilator circuits?

_____

50. How much volume will be lost in the patient circuit when the tubing compressibility is 2.5 mL/cm $H_2O$, the set volume is 500 mL, 0 PEEP, and the PIP is 25 cm $H_2O$?

51. Give two reasons why exhaled tidal volume ($V_T$) may not equal the set $V_T$ when a breath is volume cycled.
    a. _____
    b. _____

52. A large leak is detected in the ventilator system during pressure-support ventilation. How will the ventilator end inspiration?

_____

53. The ventilator cycles to expiration when the patient's exhaled gas flow drops to a certain percentage of the peak inspiratory flow rate. This describes what type of end to inspiration?

_____

54. Give a clinical scenario where a pressure-cycled ventilator could be used.

_____

_____

55. How does flow cycling occur during pressure-support ventilation?

_____

_____

_____

56. What flow is required to deliver 600 mL in 1 second with a constant gas flow?

_____

_____

57. What happens to inspiratory and expiratory times during an inflation hold?

_____

58. List three terms also used to describe an inflation hold.
   a. _____
   b. _____
   c. _____

59. Air trapping can occur following an inflation hold if

_____.

60. Define the expiratory phase.

_____

61. The pressure level from which a ventilator breath begins is called the _____.

62. The addition of a positive pressure to exhalation during mechanical ventilation is called

_____.

63. What type of ventilator assists both inspiration and expiration by pushing air into the lungs and pulling it back out at extremely high frequencies?

_____

64. A patient who is intubated and receiving mechanical ventilation is allowed to exhale. The ventilator then closes both expiratory and inspiratory valves. This maneuver is known as _____ and measures the amount of _____.

65. Increased resistance to exhalation may be caused by what devices?

_____

66. The application of pressures above ambient throughout inspiration and expiration to improve oxygenation in a spontaneously breathing patient is referred to as _____.

67. What are the two pressure sets during bilevel positive-pressure ventilation?
   a. _____
   b. _____

## CRITICAL THINKING QUESTIONS

Questions 1 through 6 refer to Figure 3.3, which shows a pressure–time curve and flow–time curve.

1. What is the limit mechanism for these breaths?

_____

2. Name the three possible modes that these graphs represent.
   a. _____
   b. _____
   c. _____

3. What is the trigger mechanism for the breaths shown?

_____

4. What is the cycling mechanism for the breaths shown?

_____

5. What is the inspiratory time? _____

6. What is the expiratory time? _____

Questions 7 through 10 refer to Figure 3.4.

7. What is the trigger variable for waveform *A*?

_____

8. What is the trigger variable for waveform *B*?

_____

9. The transairway pressure is _____.

10. What is the baseline? _____

## CASE STUDIES

### Case Study 1

You are a respiratory therapist assigned to the ICU of a local hospital and have been called to assess a patient who may require mechanical ventilation. Physical examination reveals a respiratory rate of 25, blood pressure 145/90, pulse 115, and breath sounds are bilaterally decreased, especially in the bases. The arterial blood gas reveals:

pH 7.44
$P_aCO_2$ 36 mm Hg
$P_aO_2$ 42 mm Hg
$S_aO_2$ 70%
$HCO_3^-$ 22 mEq/L
Device: a nonrebreather mask at 10 L/min
The patient's maximal inspiratory pressure is –75 cm $H_2O$, VC is 70 mL/kg, and $V_T$ is 7 mL/kg.

1. Explain the primary area of concern for this patient.

   _____

   _____

   _____

2. What is the most appropriate type of ventilatory support for this patient at this time?

   _____

   _____

The following day you return to the ICU and find this patient is receiving mechanical ventilation. Figure 3.5 shows the graphic display.

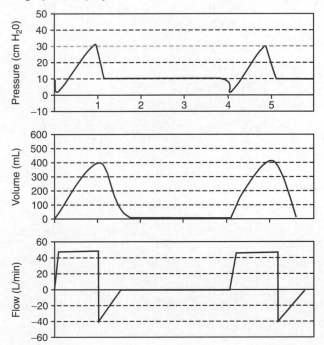

3. What type of ventilation is this patient receiving?

   _____

4. What is (are) the limiting variable(s)?

   _____

5. What trigger variable is being used at this time?

_____

In addition, you note that the patient is diaphoretic and is using accessory muscles while assisting.

6. Do any of the graphic displays give clues to the source of this patient's problem? If so, which one(s)?

_____

7. What is likely the source of this patient's problem?

_____

_____

_____

8. To alleviate this problem, what should you do?

_____

_____

## Case Study 2

A postoperative patient is being placed on a mechanical ventilator in volume-controlled ventilation.

1. What parameters need to be set by the respiratory therapist?

_____

_____

2. During mechanical ventilation, the patient's PIP is reaching 28 cm $H_2O$. At what level should the maximum safety pressure be set?

_____

3. What is the purpose of the maximum safety pressure?

_____

_____

While performing a patient-ventilator assessment, the respiratory therapist notices that although a $V_T$ of 500 mL is set, only an exhaled $V_T$ of 400 mL is being measured, and the maximum safety pressure is reached during each breath.

4. What is the most likely cause for the difference between the set and exhaled $V_T$? Explain your answer.

_____

_____

_____

5. If the maximum safety pressure was not reached on each breath and the exhaled volume was 100 mL less than the set $V_T$, what could be the possible causes?

_____

_____

## NBRC-STYLE QUESTIONS

1. A breath that is triggered, limited, and cycled by the mechanical ventilator is which of the following?
   a. Assisted
   b. Mandatory
   c. Spontaneous
   d. Synchronized

2. A breath that is triggered, controlled, and ended by the patient is which of the following?
   a. Assisted
   b. Controlled
   c. Spontaneous
   d. Synchronized

3. A breath that is patient triggered, ventilator controlled, and cycled is which of the following?
   a. Assisted
   b. Controlled
   c. Spontaneous
   d. Pressure supported

4. During pressure-controlled ventilation, the patient's airway resistance ($R_{aw}$) increases. This will cause which of the following to occur?
   a. The peak pressure will increase.
   b. The peak pressure will decrease.
   c. The delivered $V_T$ will increase.
   d. The delivered $V_T$ will decrease.

5. During volume-controlled ventilation, the patient's lung compliance improves. This will cause which of the following to occur?
   a. The peak pressure will increase.
   b. The peak pressure will decrease.
   c. The delivered $V_T$ will increase.
   d. The delivered $V_T$ will decrease.

6. During volume-controlled ventilation, which waveform remains unchanged with changes in the patient's lung characteristics?
   1. Volume–time curve
   2. Pressure–time curve
   3. Flow–time curve
   a. 1 only
   b. 2 only
   c. 1 and 3 only
   d. 2 and 3 only

7. When both pressure and volume waveforms are affected by changes in lung characteristics, which of the following variables is being controlled?
   a. Time
   b. Flow
   c. Volume
   d. Pressure

8. A high-frequency oscillator controls which of the following variables?
   a. Flow
   b. Time
   c. Volume
   d. Pressure

9. When the ventilator is time triggering and the rate is set at 20 breaths/min, the time interval between breaths is which of the following?
   a. 2 seconds
   b. 3 seconds
   c. 4 seconds
   d. 5 seconds

10. During flow triggering, the base flow is set at 5 L/min, and the ventilator triggers when it senses 3 L/min returning to its flow measuring device. The flow sensitivity setting is which of the following?
    a. 2 L/min
    b. 3 L/min
    c. 5 L/min
    d. 8 L/min

11. During pressure-support ventilation, the patient triggers the ventilator, the set pressure is reached, and the ventilator cycles at 5 seconds. What is the cause of this time cycle?
    a. A leak in the system.
    b. This is the normal setting.
    c. Increased lung compliance.
    d. Change in $R_{aw}$.

12. The most common cycling mechanism used for pressure-support ventilation is which of the following?
    a. Time
    b. Flow
    c. Volume
    d. Pressure

13. The maneuver used to measure plateau pressure is which of the following?
    a. Flow limiting
    b. Expiratory hold
    c. Inspiratory hold
    d. Pressure limiting

14. What is the transrespiratory pressure if the ventilator is set at a volume of 500 mL with a flow of 60 L/min and the patient's lung compliance is 0.75 L/cm $H_2O$ and the $R_{aw}$ is 6 cm $H_2O$/L/s?
    a. 0.12 cm $H_2O$
    b. 4.5 cm $H_2O$
    c. 6.7 cm $H_2O$
    d. 7.5 cm $H_2O$

15. What flow is needed to deliver 850 mL of volume to a patient in 0.75 second with a constant gas flow?
    a. 53 L/min
    b. 60 L/min
    c. 68 L/min
    d. 75 L/min

# 4 Establishing the Need for Mechanical Ventilation

## LEARNING OBJECTIVES

*Upon completion of this chapter, the reader will be able to do the following:*

1. Differentiate between acute respiratory failure (ARF) and respiratory insufficiency.
2. Describe three categories of disorders that may lead to respiratory insufficiency or ARF.
3. Compare normal values for the vital capacity, maximum inspiratory pressure, maximum expiratory pressure (MEP), forced expiratory volume in 1 second (FEV$_1$), peak expiratory flow, physiological dead space/tidal volume (V$_D$/V$_T$) ratio, alveolar-arterial oxygen pressure difference (P$_{[A-a]}$O$_2$), and arterial to alveolar partial pressure of oxygen (P$_a$O$_2$/P$_A$O$_2$) ratio with abnormal values that indicate the need for ventilatory support.

**KEY TEMRS CROSSWORD PUZZLE**

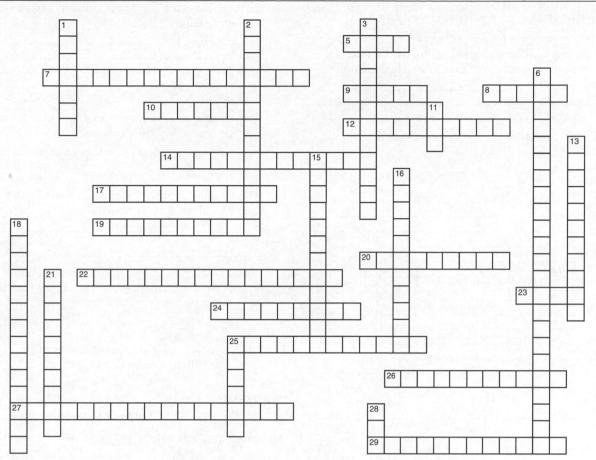

## Across

5 An indicator of airway obstruction (abbreviation)
7 Type of neuromuscular disease that causes descending paralysis
8 Condition in which perfusion of vital organs is inadequate to meet their metabolic needs
9 Breathing that has irregular periods of apnea alternating with periods of deep breathing
10 Type of respiratory failure also referred to as *lung failure*
12 Sleepiness
14 Type of neuromuscular disease that causes ascending paralysis
17 Respiratory failure referred to as *pump failure*
19 Type of hypoxemia that is resistant to treatment
20 Rapid breathing
22 Controversial treatment for a closed head wound
23 State of unconsciousness
24 State of lethargy and immobility with diminished responsiveness to stimulation
25 Above the sternum
26 Normal respiratory balance
27 Latin for acute, severe asthma (two words)
29 An abnormal breathing pattern characterized by alternating progressive hypopnea and hypoventilation ending in brief apnea (two words)

## Down

1 Pus in the pleural spacesuper
2 Measurement used to assess respiratory muscle strength (two words)
3 Device used to measure volumes at the bedside
6 Absent or inadequate respiratory activity (three words)
11 Condition characterized by alveolar flooding caused by an acute insult (abbreviation)
13 Breathing pattern characterized by abnormal movement of the thorax and the abdomen
15 Breathing pattern in which the rib cage and the abdomen do not move outward together
16 Early indicator of hypoxemia
18 Abnormal anteroposterior and lateral curvature of the spine
21 Blood in the pleural space
25 Toxic condition arising from infection
28 When increasing the lung volume, this increases (abbreviation)

**CHAPTER REVIEW QUESTIONS**

1. What is the primary purpose of ventilation?
   _____

2. List and explain the components of the three basic physiologic objectives of mechanical ventilation.
   a. _____
   b. _____
   c. _____

3. List eight clinical objectives of mechanical ventilation.
   a. _____
   b. _____
   c. _____
   d. _____
   e. _____
   f. _____
   g. _____
   h. _____

4. List ten physical signs of respiratory distress.
   a. _____
   b. _____
   c. _____
   d. _____
   e. _____
   f. _____
   g. _____
   h. _____
   i. _____
   j. _____

5. Define acute respiratory failure.

6. Clinically, what arterial blood gas (ABG) measurements indicate ARF?
   a. _____
   b. _____
   c. _____

7. List and define the two forms of acute respiratory failure and give examples of each.
   a. _____
   b. _____

8. Basic treatment for hypoxemic respiratory failure includes _____ possibly in combination with _____.

9. What does the ventilatory pump consist of?
   _____

   _____

10. List five disorders that reduce the drive to breathe.
    a. _____
    b. _____
    c. _____
    d. _____
    e. _____

11. List five disorders associated with neuromuscular function that can cause hypoventilation and possible respiratory failure.
    a. _____
    b. _____
    c. _____
    d. _____
    e. _____

12. What chest wall deformities result in increased work of breathing?
    _____

    _____

13. What pulmonary diseases cause increased airway resistance and result in increased work of breathing?

    _____

    _____

14. What should be included in an initial rapid assessment of a patient with possible respiratory failure?
    _____

    _____

15. Fill in the following chart as it relates to the conditions seen with hypoxemia and hypercapnia.

**HYPOXEMIA**

|  | Mild to Moderate | Severe |
|---|---|---|
| Respiratory findings | _____ | _____ |
| Cardiovascular findings | _____ | _____ |
| Neurologic findings | _____ | _____ |

**HYPERCAPNIA**

|  | Mild to Moderate | Severe |
|---|---|---|
| Respiratory findings | _____ | _____ |
| Cardiovascular findings | _____ | _____ |
| Neurologic findings | _____ | _____ |
| Signs | _____ | _____ |

16. What three elements are required to successfully treat a patient in acute or impending respiratory failure?
    a. _____
    b. _____
    c. _____

17. Patients with central nervous system dysfunctions may exhibit what two breathing patterns?
    a. _____
    b. _____

18. How often should a patient with a neuromuscular disorder and respiratory fatigue be monitored for changes in their respiratory status?
    _____

19. What two measurements should be used to monitor a patient with a neuromuscular disorder and respiratory fatigue to test for muscle strength? What are their critical values?

    a. _____

    b. _____

20. What limits tolerance to an increased work of breathing?

    _____

21. List three signs of increased work of breathing.

    a. _____

    b. _____

    c. _____

22. What is a normal maximum inspiratory pressure (MIP)?

    _____

23. What is another name for MIP?

    _____

24. MIP measurement stops when the lowest negative value is reached, which can take up to _____ seconds.

25. What is the normal range for vital capacity?

    _____

26. ARF is most likely present when minute ventilation exceeds _____.

27. What pulmonary function parameter can be used at the bedside to identify increased airway resistance? What measurement is considered critical?

    _____

28. An indicator of adequate airway patency and airway resistance is _____. What measurement is considered critical? _____

29. Adequate ventilation can be determined by looking at what ABG value? _____

30. The normal VD/VT range is between _____ _____ and _____ at normal tidal volumes. The critical value for this measurement is _____.

31. List three common causes of increased dead space ventilation.

    a. _____

    b. _____

    c. _____

32. Complete the following table for oxygen status assessment.

| Measurement | Normal Range | Critical Value |
| --- | --- | --- |
| $P(A-a)O_2$ | _____ | _____ |
| $P_aO_2/P_AO_2$ | _____ | _____ |
| $P_aO_2/F_IO_2$ | _____ | _____ |

33. A patient with congestive heart failure is receiving NIV. The patient is not responding well to this therapy. What action should be taken at this time?

    _____

34. What are the two key indicators of the severity of acute hypoxemic respiratory failure?

    _____

35. Based on ABG values, list five indications that suggest the need for invasive mechanical ventilation.

    a. _____

    b. _____

    c. _____

    d. _____

    e. _____

36. In what type of situation would intubation be contraindicated?

    _____

    _____

37. List three indications for NIV in an adult.

    a. _____

    b. _____

    c. _____

38. List five absolute contraindications for NIV in an adult.

    a. _____

    b. _____

    c. _____

    d. _____

    e. _____

39. A 48-year-old woman with a past medical history of congestive heart failure and hypertension is brought to the emergency department (ED) complaining of an acute onset of dyspnea. The patient has frothy pink sputum, pulse is 120 beats/min and irregular, and respirations are 26 breaths/min and labored. Breath sounds reveal bilateral basilar crackles and rhonchi. ABG results: pH 7.31, $P_aCO_2$ 48 mm Hg, $P_aO_2$ 50 mm Hg, and $S_aO_2$ 72% on a nonrebreathing mask at 10 L/min. What respiratory therapy modalities should be recommended for this patient?

    _____

    _____

    _____

    _____

    _____

40. A 79-year-old man with inoperable lung cancer develops acute severe dyspnea. The patient's pulse is 104 beats/min and regular and respirations are 24 breaths/min with accessory muscles being used. Breath sounds are decreased bilaterally in the bases. What treatment should the respiratory therapist recommend for this patient?

_____

_____

_____

_____

41. A 51-year-old woman presented to the ED complaining of shortness of breath and chest tightness for 2 days. Physical exam reveals pulse 122 beats/min and respirations 35 breaths/min with accessory muscle use. Breath sounds reveal bilateral inspiratory and expiratory wheezing with diminished breath sounds in the bases. The patient is alert and oriented but extremely anxious. ABGs reveal pH 7.22, $P_aCO_2$ 55 mm Hg, and $P_aO_2$ 51 mm Hg on room air. What course of treatment is most appropriate for this patient?

_____

_____

_____

_____

42. A 65-year-old man was admitted this morning with an exacerbation of chronic obstructive pulmonary disease (COPD). Physical exam reveals pulse 107 beats/min and regular, respirations 24 breaths/min and slightly labored, oral temperature 38.5°C, and blood pressure (BP) 141/90 mm Hg. Breath sounds are much decreased, especially in the bases. ABG results show pH 7.44, $P_aCO_2$ 33 mm Hg, $P_aO_2$ 52 mm Hg, and $HCO_3^-$ 33 mEq/L. What recommendations should the respiratory therapist make for this patient?

_____

_____

_____

43. A 23-year-old man is brought to the ED via ambulance following a bicycle accident in which he suffered head trauma. The patient is unresponsive, pulse is 112 beats/min and regular, respirations are 40 breaths/min and shallow, and breath sounds are decreased throughout. ABG reveals pH 7.21, $P_aCO_2$ 59 mm Hg, and $P_aO_2$ 50 mm Hg on a nasal cannula at 6 L/min. What recommendations should the respiratory therapist make for this patient?

_____

_____

_____

_____

44. Calculate the arterial oxygen content for a patient with the following ABG results: pH 7.44, $P_aCO_2$ 44 mm Hg, $P_aO_2$ 59 mm Hg, $S_aO_2$ 91%, $F_IO_2$ 0.21, hemoglobin (Hb) 12 g/dL. Show all work.

_____

_____

_____

45. Calculate the arterial oxygen content for a patient with the following ABG results: pH 7.34, $P_aCO_2$ 22 mm Hg, $P_aO_2$ 58 mm Hg, $S_aO_2$ 90%, Hb 8 g/dL. Show all work.

_____

_____

_____

46. Calculate the arterial oxygen content for a patient with the following ABG results: pH 7.36, $P_aCO_2$ 59 mm Hg, $P_aO_2$ 48 mm Hg, $S_aO_2$ 79%, Hb 17 g/dL. Show all work.

_____

_____

_____

47. Calculate the $P(A - a)O_2$ for a patient with the following ABG results: pH 7.31, $P_aCO_2$ 48 mm Hg, $P_aO_2$ 50 mm Hg, $S_aO_2$ 72% on a nonrebreathing mask at 12 L/min. (Assume the nonrebreathing mask is delivering approximately 70% oxygen.) Show all work.

_____

_____

_____

_____

48. Calculate the arterial/alveolar $PO_2$ for the patient in Question 47. What does this mean, and is this a critical value?

_____

_____

49. Calculate the $P_aO_2/F_IO_2$ for the patient in Question 47. (Assume the nonrebreathing mask is delivering approximately 70% oxygen.) Is this a critical value?

_____

_____

50. Calculate the $P(A - a)O_2$ for the patient with the following ABG results: pH 7.22, $P_aCO_2$ 55 mm Hg, $P_aO_2$ 51 mm Hg on room air. Is this value an indication for mechanical ventilation?

_____

_____

_____

51. Calculate the arterial/alveolar $PO_2$ for the patient in Question 50. Is this a critical value?

_____

_____

52. Calculate the $P_aO_2/F_IO_2$ for the patient in Question 50. Is this a critical value?

_____

_____

_____

_____

## CRITICAL THINKING QUESTIONS

1. You are called to the ED to perform a cardiopulmonary assessment of a patient who has just been brought in following a motor vehicle accident. What would be your rapid physical assessment?

_____

_____

_____

_____

2. Following your initial physical assessment of the patient in Question 1, what diagnostic evaluations should be done to assess the need for mechanical ventilation?

_____

_____

3. Describe how a patient in respiratory distress might look.

_____

_____

4. Discuss the difference in clinical presentation between a patient needing oxygen therapy only and one who needs mechanical ventilation.

_____

_____

_____

_____

## CASE STUDIES

### Case Study 1

A 35-year-old male, with a history of asthma, was admitted from the ED to the Intensive Care Unit (ICU). The patient is alert, oriented, extremely anxious, sitting up, and leaning on the bedside tray table. Physical examination reveals pulse 142 beats/min, BP 178/86 mm Hg, oral temperature 37.9°C, and respirations 33 breaths/min and labored. Chest auscultation reveals significantly decreased breath sounds throughout with slight wheezing on exhalation. ABG results on 40% air entrainment mask include the following:

pH 7.33
$P_aCO_2$ 44 mm Hg
$P_aO_2$ 48 mm Hg

$S_aO_2$ 79%
$HCO_3^-$ 22 mEq/L
Hb 14.8 g/dL
The peak expiratory flow reading is 70 L/min following three consecutive bronchodilator treatments.

1. What is the most likely cause of the patient's tachycardia?

_____

2. Using oxygenation indicators, explain the oxygenation status of this patient. (Assume $P_B$ is 760.)

_____

_____

3. Although this patient's $P_aCO_2$ is within normal limits, why is it significant in this case?

_____

_____

4. What respiratory care treatment should be suggested for this patient?

_____

_____

_____

_____

## Case Study 2

A 46-year-old female was admitted to the ICU a few hours ago with an acute exacerbation of myasthenia gravis. She is alert and oriented, pulse is 102 beats/min and regular, BP is 140/75 mm Hg, oral temperature is 37.4°C, and respirations are 30 breaths/min and very shallow. Breath sounds are decreased throughout. She cannot cough. The patient is complaining of weakness and difficulty swallowing. ABGs on room air reveal pH 7.36, $P_aCO_2$ 38 mm Hg, $P_aO_2$ 60 mm Hg, $S_aO_2$ 90%, $HCO_3^-$ 20 mEq/L, and Hb 12.6 g/dL. The maximum inspiratory pressure is 30 cm $H_2O$.

1. What is this patient's oxygenation status? Explain your answer.

_____

_____

_____

2. Evaluate this patient's ventilatory status.

_____

_____

_____

3. What treatment or monitoring recommendations should be made for this patient?

_____

_____

_____

## Case Study 3

A 76-year-old female presents to the ED in severe respiratory failure due to COPD. Her ABG results show pH 7.15, $P_aCO_2$ 90 mm Hg, $P_aO_2$ 43 mm Hg, $HCO_3^-$ 29 mEq/L, $S_aO_2$ 52% on $F_IO_2$ 0.4, and CPAP 5 cm $H_2O$. The patient appears drowsy.

1. What is this patient's oxygenation status? Explain your answer.

2. Evaluate this patient's ventilatory status.

3. What treatment or monitoring recommendations should be made for this patient?

## NBRC-STYLE QUESTIONS

1. A 43-year-old male was admitted last night with a stab wound to the right anterior thorax. The wound was repaired in surgery. Currently the patient is alert and continuously tries to remove his oxygen mask. He is in the ICU and has a chest tube in his right hemithorax. Vital signs show pulse 120 beats/min, respirations 36 breaths/min and shallow, BP 148/90 mm Hg, and oral temperature 38° C. Breath sounds are decreased over the right base, and chest expansion is decreased over the right side. The patient is not coughing. ABG results reveal pH 7.48, $P_aCO_2$ 26 mm Hg, $P_aO_2$ 66 mm Hg, $S_aO_2$ 94%, $HCO_3^-$ 19 mEq/L, $F_IO_2$ 0.55 (via an air entrainment mask), and Hb 11.4. Which of the following is the most appropriate action to take at this time?
   a. Increase the $F_IO_2$ to 0.5.
   b. Place the patient on bilevel positive airway pressure.
   c. Administer albuterol via a small volume nebulizer.
   d. Intubate and mechanically ventilate with an $F_IO_2$ of 1.0.

2. Which of the following characterizes hypercapnic respiratory failure?
   1. Lower than normal $P_aO_2$
   2. Alveolar hypoventilation
   3. Higher than normal $P_aCO_2$
   4. Increased $P_AO_2 - P_aO_2$
   a. 1 and 2 only
   b. 1, 2, and 3 only
   c. 2 and 3 only
   d. 2, 3, and 4 only

3. The underlying physiological process leading to pure hypercapnic respiratory failure is which of the following?
   a. Low V/Q ratio
   b. Diffusion impairment
   c. Intrapulmonary shunting
   d. Alveolar hypoventilation

4. A 65-year-old male presents to the ED complaining of increasing shortness of breath over the past 3 days and appears to be in moderate respiratory distress. He has a 100-pack-year smoking history. Vital signs are heart rate 115 beats/min, respiratory rate 32 breaths/min, BP 170/95 mm Hg, mild expiratory wheezing in his bases, and temperature 100° F oral. His ABG values on nasal cannula 3 L/min are pH 7.30, $P_aCO_2$ 70 mm Hg, $P_aO_2$ 48 mm Hg, $S_aO_2$ 67%, and $HCO_3^-$ 35 mEq/L. The most appropriate treatment at this time is to initiate which of the following?
   a. Bronchodilator therapy
   b. Air entrainment mask at 35%
   c. Intubation and mechanical ventilation
   d. Noninvasive positive pressure ventilation

5. A 55-year-old female with a history of chronic congestive heart failure and extreme obesity presents to the ED. She is alert but disoriented. Vital signs show pulse 143 beats/min, BP 145/94 mm Hg, oral temperature 37° C, and respirations 28 breaths/min shallow and labored. She has no cough. Breath sounds are decreased throughout with bilateral inspiratory coarse crackles. Electrocardiogram shows sinus tachycardia with a widened QRS complex and an occasional premature ventricular contraction. Her ABGs on a 50% air entrainment mask are pH 7.30, $P_aCO_2$ 51 mm Hg, $P_aO_2$ 50 mm Hg, $S_aO_2$ 85%, and $HCO_3^-$ 24 mEq/L. Which of the following should the respiratory therapist should recommend at this time?
   a. Nonrebreathing mask
   b. CPAP
   c. Intubation and mechanical ventilation
   d. Bilevel noninvasive positive pressure ventilation

6. An 18-year-old man is brought to the ED via ambulance following a serious bicycle crash with witnesses stating the patient was not wearing a helmet. The patient is unconscious and semiresponsive with a Glasgow Coma Score of 1/1/4 totaling 6. Vital signs show pulse 110 beats/min and regular, BP 96/55 mm Hg, oral temperature 36.6° C, and respirations 38 breaths/min and shallow with no cough. Chest auscultation reveals decreased breath sounds throughout. ABG results on a simple mask at 6 L/min are pH 7.22, $P_aCO_2$ 58 mm Hg, $P_aO_2$ 52 mm Hg, $S_aO_2$ 76%, and $HCO_3^-$ 22 mEq/L. Based on these findings the respiratory therapist should initiate which of the following?
   a. Nonrebreathing mask
   b. CPAP
   c. Intubation and mechanical ventilation
   d. Noninvasive positive pressure ventilation

7. A 135-pound patient with Guillain-Barré has been monitored in the ICU by the respiratory therapist over the past 6 hours. Both MIPs and vital capacity (VC) values have been recorded as follows:

| Time | MIP | VC |
| --- | --- | --- |
| 7:00 AM | −40 cm $H_2O$ | 3.1 L |
| 9:15 AM | −35 cm $H_2O$ | 2.8 L |
| 11:25 AM | −25 cm $H_2O$ | 1.5 L |
| 1:10 PM | −15 cm $H_2O$ | 0.64 L |

Following the last assessment at 1:10 PM, what therapeutic intervention should the respiratory therapist recommend?
   a. 50% air entrainment mask
   b. CPAP
   c. Intubation and mechanical ventilation
   d. Noninvasive positive pressure ventilation

8. A 40-year-old woman presents to the ED with a 2-day history of dyspnea; productive cough with thick, green sputum; fever; and chills. The respiratory therapist's assessment reveals the following: pulse 105 beats/min, respirations 30 breaths/min, BP 132/84 mm Hg, oral temperature 39°C, decreased chest excursion of the right, and dull percussion over the right base. Chest auscultation indicates coarse crackles and wheezes over the right base. ABG results on room air reveal pH 7.35, $P_aCO_2$ 31 mm Hg, $P_aO_2$ 72 mm Hg, $S_aO_2$ 88%, and $HCO_3^-$ 24 mEq/L. The respiratory therapist should recommend which of the following?
   a. Nasal cannula at 4 L/min
   b. Continuous aerosol with 30% oxygen
   c. CPAP
   d. Noninvasive positive pressure ventilation

9. Which of the following conditions demonstrates the need for intubation and mechanical ventilation?
   a. Moderate hypoxemia
   b. ARF
   c. Chronic respiratory failure
   d. Hypoxic respiratory failure

10. A disorder that may cause hypercapnic respiratory failure because of increased work of breathing includes which of the following?
   a. Asthma
   b. Botulism
   c. Metabolic acidosis
   d. Cerebral hemorrhage

# 5 Selecting the Ventilator and the Mode

*On completion of this chapter, the reader will be able to do the following:*

1. Select an appropriate mechanical ventilator, breath type, and mode of ventilation based on clinical findings derived from patient assessment data.
2. Describe how continuous positive airway pressure (CPAP) and noninvasive positive pressure ventilation (NIV) can be used in the management of patients with various cardiopulmonary disorders.
3. Discuss the advantages and disadvantages of volume-controlled and pressure-controlled ventilation.
4. Explain the differences in function among continuous mandatory ventilation, spontaneous ventilation, and intermittent mandatory ventilation.
5. Describe the functions of the *trigger, cycle,* and *limit* variables as they are used in volume-controlled continuous mandatory ventilation, pressure-controlled continuous mandatory ventilation, volume-controlled intermittent mandatory ventilation, pressure-controlled intermittent mandatory ventilation, and pressure support ventilation.
6. Define each of the following terms: *pressure augmentation, pressure-regulated volume control, volume support, mandatory minute ventilation, airway pressure release ventilation, bilevel positive airway pressure,* and *proportional assist ventilation.*

## KEY TERMS CROSSWORD PUZZLE

**Across**

3 Over ventilation in the CMV mode can cause this (two words)
5 A mode of ventilation that uses two levels of continuous positive airway pressure (CPAP) (abbreviation)
9 When the patient controls the timing and the tidal volume (two words)
11 Inverse ventilation with pressure control (abbreviation)
12 Type of control variable
13 Mode of ventilation with only time-triggered breaths (two words)
14 The ventilator supplies all the energy necessary to maintain alveolar ventilation (three words)
15 Occurs when the patient and the ventilator are not working together

**Down**

1 Mode of ventilation where all breaths are mandatory and can be volume or pressure targeted (abbreviation)
2 Type of ventilatory support where the patient is participating in the work of breathing (WOB)
4 Patient-triggered volume or pressure-targeted ventilation (hyphenated word)
6 A mode that supports the spontaneously breathing patient to help reduce the WOB (two words)
7 Type of breath where the timing and/or the tidal volume is controlled by the ventilator
8 Guarantees a specific volume delivery (two words)
9 The ventilator setting used to determine the ventilator response to the patient's inspiratory effort
10 A cross between mandatory and spontaneous breaths

**CHAPTER REVIEW QUESTIONS**

1. List seven questions that the clinician should ask when determining the appropriate ventilator and mode of ventilation.

    a. _____

    b. _____

    c. _____

    d. _____

    e. _____

    f. _____

    g. _____

2. Match the appropriate ventilation support type with the appropriate ventilator connection or interface (there may be more than one answer):

    _____ Negative pressure       A. Oral endotracheal
            ventilation                  tube
    _____ CPAP                     B. Nasal mask
    _____ Positive pressure        C. Face mask
            ventilation              D. Chest cuirass
    _____ Noninvasive positive     E. Tracheostomy
            pressure ventilation         tube

3. CPAP is commonly used in the hospital setting as a method to _____, while in the home-care setting it is typically used when treating _____.

4. Acute-on-chronic respiratory failure is most often treated with which type of noninvasive positive-pressure ventilation (NIV)?

5. Name a type of ventilation that reduces the requirements for heavy patient sedation.

    _____

6. List five disorders that are sometimes managed with NIV.

    a. _____

    b. _____

    c. _____

    d. _____

    e. _____

7. List both advantages and disadvantages of NIV in a patient with acute respiratory failure.

    **Advantage**                **Disadvantage**

    _____        _____

    _____        _____

    _____        _____

    _____        _____

    _____        _____

8. Define the terms *full ventilatory support* and *partial ventilatory support*.

    _____

    _____

    _____

9. The typical minimum ventilatory rate setting for a patient receiving full ventilatory support is considered _____ breaths/min.

10. Partial ventilatory support typically uses set machine rates of lower than _____ breaths/min with the patient participating in the WOB to help maintain effective alveolar ventilation.

11. What type of ventilatory support would you consider using when your patient has acute ventilatory failure from ventilatory muscle fatigue or a high WOB? Why?

    _____

    _____

    _____

12. List and explain the three types of breath delivery.

    a. _____

    b. _____

    c. _____

13. What is the primary advantage of volume-controlled ventilation?

    _____

14. What is the main disadvantage of volume-controlled ventilation?

    _____

15. During volume-control ventilation, a patient develops acute bronchospasm. What will happen to (a) the peak inspiratory pressure? Why? What will happen to (b) the amount of volume delivered to the patient? Why?

    a. _____

    _____

    b. _____

    _____

16. A patient experiencing acute bronchospasm receives an adrenergic bronchodilator. If the bronchodilator is effective, the peak inspiratory pressure is expected to _____. Why?

    _____

17. When targeting pressure as the control variable, what will vary with changing lung characteristics?

    _____

18. What are three advantages of pressure-control ventilation (PCV)?

    a. _____

    b. _____

    c. _____

19. What are three disadvantages of PCV?

    a. _____

    b. _____

    c. _____

20. When a patient's lung compliance worsens during PCV, what will happen to the tidal volume being delivered?

    _____

21. What are the three types of breath delivery timing or sequence available on current intensive care unit (ICU) ventilators? Briefly describe each.

    a. _____

    b. _____

    c. _____

22. What three characteristics determine the mode of ventilation?

    a. _____

    b. _____

    c. _____

23. List the five basic modes of ventilation.

    a. _____

    b. _____

    c. _____

    d. _____

    e. _____

24. How should clinicians differentiate between controlled and assisted ventilation?

    _____

25. Give a clinical situation where assist-controlled ventilation is appropriate?

    _____

    _____

    _____

26. What happens when the clinician inappropriately sets ventilator sensitivity?

    _____

    _____

27. What two triggers can begin inspiration in patient-triggered assisted ventilation?

    a. _____

    b. _____

28. Studies have shown that VC-CMV may actually increase the patient's WOB by _____%. How is this observed in the clinical setting? How is this corrected?

    _____

29. What settings are typically set by the clinician in PC-CMV?

    _____

    _____

30. What determines the tidal volume delivered in PC-CMV?

    _____

31. What flow-curve type has been shown to improve gas distribution and allow the patient to vary inspiratory gas flow during spontaneous breathing efforts?

    _____

32. A safety mechanism to avoid excessive system pressure is the _____ and is set at about _____ above the set pressure level and will cause _____ to end when reached.

33. Describe a clinical scenario where pressure controlled inverse ratio ventilation (PC-IRV) would be appropriate?

    _____

    _____

34. Explain how IMV differs from CMV?

    _____

    _____

    _____

35. Fill in the table below regarding the advantages, risks, and disadvantages of CMV and IMV.

| Mode | Advantages | Risks and Disadvantages |
|---|---|---|
| VC-CMV or PC-CMV | _____ _____ _____ _____ _____ _____ _____ _____ _____ _____ _____ _____ _____ _____ _____ _____ _____ | _____ _____ _____ _____ _____ _____ _____ _____ _____ _____ _____ _____ _____ _____ _____ _____ _____ |
| VC-IMV or PC-IMV | _____ _____ _____ _____ _____ _____ _____ _____ _____ _____ _____ _____ _____ _____ _____ _____ _____ | _____ _____ _____ _____ _____ _____ _____ _____ _____ _____ _____ _____ _____ _____ _____ _____ _____ |

36. What is the goal when choosing IMV mode for a patient?

_____

37. What are the three basic means of providing support for continuous spontaneous breathing during mechanical ventilation?

a. _____

b. _____

c. _____

38. Briefly describe a spontaneous breathing trial.

_____

39. What patient characteristics are necessary for PSV to be successful?

_____

_____

40. What ventilator parameters are set by the clinician in PSV? What parameters does the patient establish?

_____

41. What determines tidal volume in PSV?

_____

_____

42. What situation can cause the ventilator in the PSV mode to time cycle?

_____

43. Define the term *rise time*.

_____

44. Inspiration is _____ cycled in PSV.

45. Give a clinical scenario where patients may require a shorter inspiratory time.

_____

46. What pressure levels does a clinician set in bilevel pressure assist?

_____

47. What patient variables can end inspiration in the bilevel pressure-assist mode?

_____

48. What patient characteristic can influence the specific time and pressure limits used during PSV?

_____

49. Explain how pressure augmentation ($P_{Aug}$) works? What is an alternate term used to describe $P_{(aug)}$?

_____

_____

_____

50. In $P_{Aug}$, if the set volume is achieved prior to flow cycling, what will happen to the breath?

_____

51. In $P_{Aug}$, if the set volume is not reached before flow drops to the set level, how will the ventilator respond?

_____

_____

52. Describe a clinical scenario where a patient can receive more volume than is set by the clinician in $P_{Aug}$?

_____

_____

_____

53. Describe PRVC in terms of trigger, limit, and cycle.

_____

54. Fill in the table below regarding the different proprietary names given to PRVC.

| Ventilator | PRVC name |
|---|---|
| CareFusion Avea | • |
| Covidien PB 840 and PB980 | • |
| Hamilton G5 | • |
| Dräger Evita Infinity | • |
| Servo-I | • |

55. Generally, at what pressure will a ventilator alarm while in the PRVC mode if the upper pressure limit is set at 40 cm $H_2O$ and the tidal volume is set at 600 mL?

_____

_____

56. Describe volume-support ventilation (VSV) in terms of trigger, limit, and cycle.

_____

_____

_____

57. What is the difference between PRVC and VSV?

_____

_____

_____

58. Define MMV.

_____

_____

_____

59. Describe adaptive support ventilation (ASV)?

_____

_____

_____

60. The mode of ventilation that requires two levels of CPAP and allows the patient to breath spontaneously at both levels is known as

_____.

61. The optimum duration of the release time for the mode mentioned in Question 60 is a function of the _____ of the respiratory system.

62. APRV was originally intended to ventilate patients with _____.

63. With PAV, what three variables are proportional to the patient's spontaneous effort?

_____

64. In PAV mode, what two factors determine the amount of pressure produced by the ventilator?

   a. _____

   b. _____

65. What are the advantages and disadvantages of PAV?

_____

_____

_____

## CRITICAL THINKING QUESTIONS

1. A patient is waking up following surgery and is currently receiving mechanical ventilation in the PC-CMV mode. During rounds, the respiratory therapist observes the patient's use of accessory muscles, diaphoresis, patient-ventilator asynchrony, and no assisted breaths. What is the most probable source of this patient's clinical appearance? How can this be corrected?

_____

_____

_____

_____

2. If a patient's ventilatory drive increases during the use of VC-CMV, what changes will occur to the patient's acid–base balance? What can be done to regulate this?

_____

_____

_____

3. Which mode of ventilation would a home-care patient with central sleep apnea benefit from and why?

_____

_____

_____

_____

_____

4. Match the patient condition with a ventilator mode most likely to benefit the patient.

**Patient with the following:**

_____ (1) Intubated with quadriplegia from a spinal cord injury

_____ (2) Intubated with acute respiratory distress syndrome

_____ (3) Obstructive sleep apnea in the homecare setting

_____ (4) Intubated with spontaneous breathing with acute lung injury

_____ (5) Intubated with consistent spontaneous respiratory pattern

_____ (6) Nonintubated spontaneously breathing with refractory hypoxemia

_____ (7) Intubated with drug overdose

**Would benefit from this ventilator mode:**

a. Nasal mask CPAP
b. CPAP through ventilator
c. Pressure support
d. VC-CMV
e. PC-CMV with positive end-expiratory pressure (PEEP)

## CASE STUDIES

### Case Study 1

In the ICU, the respiratory therapist approaches a patient receiving mechanical ventilation. The ventilator monitor shows the following scalar.

1. What mode of ventilation is the ventilator set to deliver?

   _____

2. What is the inspiratory time for the mechanical breaths?

   _____

3. What is the ventilator expiratory time?

   _____

### Case Study 2

*A 6-foot 3-inch male patient who was involved in a motor vehicle crash (MVC) arrives in* the emergency department with chest and facial injuries. Because of the nature of the facial injuries, he is intubated with a size 8.0 mm endotracheal tube. Following resuscitative measures, he is transferred to the ICU.

1. What type of ventilator support would this patient require initially?

   _____

2. What ventilator mode would you use when this patient wakes, has the desire to breathe spontaneously, and has a $P_aO_2$ of 58 mm Hg with the $F_IO_2$ set at 0.50?

   _____

### Case Study 3

1. What mode of ventilation does Figure 5.1 represent?

   _____

2. Identify the issue with this pressure tracing.

   _____

3. What can be done to resolve the identified problem?

   _____

## NBRC-STYLE QUESTIONS

1. When switching from the CMV mode to the IMV mode to facilitate weaning from mechanical ventilation, which of the following could be used, in addition to IMV, to assist in this process?
   a. ASV
   b. PSV
   c. PAV
   d. APRV

2. A post-thoracic surgery patient currently receiving mechanical ventilation on VC-CMV with 60% oxygen has the following arterial blood gas (ABG): pH 7.45, $P_aCO_2$ 36 mm Hg, $P_aO_2$ 68 mm Hg. The patient's peak inspiratory pressures are averaging 55 cm $H_2O$. The ventilator mode that is most appropriate at this time is which of the following?
   a. PSV
   b. VC-IMV with PEEP
   c. PC-CMV with PEEP
   d. MMV

3. A 38-year-old female suffered a deceleration injury in an MVC. She is alert and oriented but in respiratory distress. A portion of the patient's right anterior chest wall is moving in a paradoxical motion. Breath sounds are decreased on the right and the trachea is midline and no pneumothorax was detected. ABG data reveal pH 7.48, $P_aCO_2$ 31 mm Hg, $P_aO_2$ 63 mm Hg, and $HCO_3^-$ 24 mEq/L. The respiratory therapist should recommend which of the following therapies for this patient at this time?
   a. Mask CPAP with supplemental oxygen
   b. Intubate and use VC-CMV with PEEP
   c. NIV with supplemental oxygen
   d. Intubate and use PCIRV

4. The physician requests that the respiratory therapist make a recommendation for a patient with postpolio complaints of increasing daytime weakness. Her VC is 12 mL/kg and maximal inspiratory pressure is −32 cm $H_2O$. Her ABG on room air reveals pH 7.38, $P_aCO_2$ 46 mm Hg, $P_aO_2$ 74 mm Hg, and $HCO_3^-$ 24 mEq/L. The respiratory therapist should suggest which of the following?
   a. Tracheostomy with PSV
   b. Tracheostomy with VC-CMV
   c. BiPAP via nasal mask at night
   d. Full face mask CPAP with supplemental oxygen

5. During a pressure-triggered breath in VC-CMV, the pressure-time curve on the graphic display does not rise smoothly and appears to be somewhat concave in appearance. This indicates which of the following?
   a. Flow rate is inadequate.
   b. Rise time is set too slow.
   c. Overshoot on the pressure.
   d. Inspiratory time is too short.

6. Every breath from the ventilator is time or patient triggered, pressure targeted (limited), and time cycled. This describes which of the following ventilator modes?
   a. $P_{Aug}$
   b. APRV
   c. PCV
   d. VC-IMV

7. Pressure augmentation ($P_{Aug}$) may be beneficial for mechanically ventilated patients with which of the following?
   1. Noncardiogenic pulmonary edema
   2. Acute Respiratory Distress Syndrome
   3. Postoperative upper abdominal surgery
   4. Receiving heavy sedation and paralyzing agents
   a. 1 and 2 only
   b. 1 and 3 only
   c. 2 and 4 only
   d. 3 and 4 only

8. The ventilator mode that allows the patient to breathe spontaneously at two levels of positive pressure is known as which of the following?
   a. CPAP
   b. $P_{Aug}$
   c. PRVC
   d. APRV

9. A patient is intubated and on PSV. The respiratory therapist notices that the inspiratory time has increased from 1 second to 2 seconds consistently on every breath since last ventilator rounds. What should be the first action the respiratory therapist should do to correct the problem?
   a. Change to the IMV mode
   b. Check the endotracheal tube cuff pressure
   c. Increase the inspiratory flow setting
   d. Suction and lavage the patient's airway

10. When the lung compliance decreases while a patient is receiving mechanical ventilation with PCV, which of the following will occur?
    a. Peak pressure will increase.
    b. Peak pressure will decrease.
    c. Tidal volume will increase.
    d. Tidal volume will decrease.

# 6 Initial Ventilator Settings

*On completion of this chapter, the reader will be able to do the following:*

1. Calculate tubing compliance.
2. Determine the volume loss caused by tubing compliance.
3. Calculate the minute ventilation given a patient's respiratory rate and tidal volume.
4. Calculate the total cycle time, inspiratory time, expiratory time, flow in liters per second, and inspiratory-to-expiratory ratios given the necessary patient data.
5. Select an appropriate flow rate and pattern.
6. Calculate the initial minute ventilation, tidal volume, and rate for a patient placed on volume-controlled continuous mandatory ventilation based on the patient's sex, height, and ideal body weight.
7. Identify the source of the problem when an inspiratory pause cannot be measured.
8. Choose an appropriate initial mode of mechanical ventilation, and determine the expired minute ventilation, tidal volume, respiratory frequency, and positive end-expiratory pressure settings based on the patient's lung pathology, body temperature, metabolic rate, altitude, and acid–base balance.
9. Evaluate the response in the peak inspiratory pressure and plateau pressure when the flow waveform is changed.
10. Recommend the selection and initial settings for the various modes of pressure ventilation, including bilevel positive airway pressure, pressure support ventilation, pressure-controlled ventilation, and Servo-controlled (dual modes) ventilation.
11. Identify a patient-ventilator problem when using pressure support ventilation from a pressure–time graph.
12. Measure the plateau pressure using pressure–time and flow–time waveforms during pressure-controlled mechanical ventilation.
13. List the possible causes for a change in pressure during pressure-regulated volume control.
14. Identify the mode of ventilation based on the trigger, target, and cycle criteria.

**KEY TERMS CROSSWORD PUZZLE**

## Across

1  Too much pressure in the alveoli can cause this
3  The abbreviation for a pressure-limited, time-cycled mode that uses the set tidal volume as a feedback control
7  Airway resistance multiplied by lung compliance is one _____ (two words)
8  The type of ventilation used to augment spontaneous breathing in patients with artificial airways (abbreviation)
10  The name of the type of flow waveform that represents the tapered flow at the end of the inspiratory phase
11  A type of flow pattern created by a progressive increase in flow during inspiration
12  The chart used to determine body surface area (BSA)
14  The type of volume that is lost in the patient circuit
17  The Dräger V500 calls its volume support by this name
18  The brand of ventilator that has no flow waveform selector or peak flow control
19  The type of flow waveform that occurs naturally in pressure ventilation

## Down

2  On the Hamilton G5 ventilator, PRVC is called _____ pressure ventilation
4  To calculate how much volume is lost in the patient circuit tubing, _____ must be known
5  One entire breathing cycle (abbreviation)
6  The type of pause used to measure plateau pressure
9  Adding tubing to the patient's endotracheal tube will add this type of dead space
10  A constant flow pattern produces this type of flow waveform
11  Air trapping is measured as this
13  The amount of inspiratory time required for the ventilator to reach the set pressure at the beginning of inspiration (two words)
15  The nomogram used to obtain ventilator settings
16  A purely spontaneous mode in which the operator sets the ventilator sensitivity, tidal volume, and upper pressure limit (abbreviation)

## CHAPTER REVIEW QUESTIONS

1. What is the primary goal of mechanical ventilation?

2. In a healthy person, what are the typical oxygen consumption and carbon dioxide consumption? What is the abbreviation used for each?

3. In humans, what two measurements is metabolic rate directly related?

4. List eight parameters to consider when setting a patient up for assist-control volume-controlled ventilation.

a. _____    e. _____
b. _____    f. _____
c. _____    g. _____
d. _____    h. _____

Questions 5 through 7 refer to Figure 6.1.

5. Find the BSA for a person who weighs 200 pounds and is 6 feet 2 inches tall.

   _____

6. Find the BSA for a person who weighs 75 kg and is 155 cm tall.

   _____

7. Find the BSA for a person who weighs 178 pounds and is 5 feet 7 inches tall.

   _____

Questions 8 through 11: Calculate minute ventilation for the following individuals.

| Question | Gender | BSA | Body Temp. | Comment | Minute Ventilation |
|---|---|---|---|---|---|
| 8. | F | 1.6 m$^2$ | 39° C | N/A | _____ |
| 9. | M | 2.8 m$^2$ | 37° C | 6000 ft above sea level | _____ |
| 10. | M | 2.3 m$^2$ | 101° F | N/A | _____ |
| 11. | F | 1.9 m$^2$ | 98.6° F | Metabolic acidosis | _____ |

12. The initial tidal volume setting for adults should be within what range?

    _____

13. The initial tidal volume setting for infants and children should be within what range?

    _____

14. The estimated $V_T$ range for a female patient who has an IBW of 50 kg is _____.

15. The estimated $V_T$ range for a male patient with an IBW of 90 kg is _____.

16. What is the normal $V_T$ range for a spontaneously breathing patient?

    _____

17. What is the normal range for the respiratory rate in a spontaneously breathing patient?

    _____

18. Recommend the initial tidal volume, respiratory rate, and minute ventilation for a 5-foot 2-inch-tall female who has just arrived in the postoperative care unit.

    _____

    _____

    _____

19. Recommend the initial tidal volume, respiratory rate, and minute ventilation for a 71-inch-tall male with chronic obstructive pulmonary disease (COPD).

    _____

    _____

    _____

20. Recommend the initial tidal volume, respiratory rate, and minute ventilation for a 69-inch-tall male with pulmonary fibrosis.

    _____

    _____

    _____

21. Calculate and fill in the missing information.

| Tidal Volume | Respiratory Rate | Minute Ventilation |
|---|---|---|
| a. 750 mL | 12 breaths/min | _____ |
| b. 580 mL | 10 breaths/min | _____ |
| c. _____ | 15 breaths/min | 6.9 L/min |
| d. _____ | 20 breaths/min | 8.3 L/min |
| e. 460 mL | _____ | 5.2 L/min |
| f. 660 mL | _____ | 9.5 L/min |

22. Calculate the total cycle time (TCT) for the following frequencies (e.g., rate setting).
    a. 30 breaths/min _____
    b. 15 breaths/min _____
    c. 12 breaths/min _____
    d. 10 breaths/min _____

23. Use the corresponding frequencies in Question 22 to calculate the expiratory time ($T_E$) for each of the given inspiratory times ($T_I$).
    a. $T_I$ = 1 second _____
    b. $T_I$ = 0.75 second _____
    c. $T_I$ = 1.25 seconds _____
    d. $T_I$ = 2 seconds _____

24. Use the corresponding information from Question 23 to determine the I:E ratios.
    a. _____
    b. _____
    c. _____
    d. _____

25. Calculate the $T_I$, $T_E$, and TCT given an I:E ratio of 1:3 and rate = 12 beats/min.

    _____

    _____

    _____

26. Calculate the $T_I$, $T_E$, and TCT given an I:E ratio of 1:2 and rate = 25 beats/min.

    _____

    _____

    _____

27. Calculate the $V_T$ given $T_I$ = 1 second and flow of 50 L/min.

    _____

    _____

    _____

28. Calculate the $T_I$ given $V_T$ = 700 mL and flow of 50 L/min.

    _____

    _____

    _____

29. Increasing the set flow rate while ventilating an apneic patient in VC-CMV will cause the $T_I$ to _____, the PIP to _____, and the gas distribution to _____.

30. What are the guidelines for setting $T_I$, I:E ratio, and flow rates during CMV?
    _____

31. The type of flow waveform pattern created by pressure ventilation is

_____ .

32. The flow waveform that creates the highest PIP during volume ventilation, when the $R_{aw}$ is elevated, is

_____

33. The flow waveform(s) most appropriate for normal lungs is (are) _____ .

34. Why is a descending flow pattern beneficial for patients with hypoxemia and low lung compliance?

_____

_____

_____

35. What is an inspiratory pause most frequently used to determine?

_____

36. The respiratory therapist attempts to measure the plateau pressure by adding a 1-second inspiratory pause. The set VC-CMV rate is 12, the current rate is 20, and the plateau pressure is unattainable. What is the most likely cause of this problem?

_____

_____

37. The pressure ventilation modes that have time triggering include

_____ .

38. The pressure ventilation modes that allow for patient triggering include

_____ .

39. Flow cycling is used by which pressure ventilation modes?

_____

40. Time cycling is used by which pressure ventilation modes?

_____

41. What are the advantages and disadvantages of using pressure ventilation?

_____

_____

_____

_____

42. Explain the concept of using low PEEP levels for patients with COPD.

_____

_____

_____

43. During pressure ventilation, how is tidal volume established?

_____

44. A patient on PC-CMV has a PIP setting of 18 cm $H_2O$. The $V_T$ is measured as 400 mL. The desired $V_T$ is 750 mL. How should the pressure be adjusted to achieve the desired $V_T$?

_____

_____

_____

45. A patient on PC-CMV has a set PIP of 14 cm $H_2O$. The exhaled $V_T$ measured is 550 mL. The desired exhaled $V_T$ is 800 mL. How should the pressure be adjusted to achieve the desired volume?

_____

_____

_____

46. What formula can be used to estimate the level of pressure support needed for a patient?

_____

_____

_____

47. During VC-CMV, the settings are as follows: f = 12 breaths/min and $V_T$ = 600 mL. The patient's PIP was measured at 28 cm $H_2O$ with a $P_{plat}$ of 20 cm $H_2O$. The patient is now ready for VC-intermittent mandatory ventilation (IMV) with pressure support. Recommend an appropriate level to start this patient's pressure support during this mode of ventilation.

_____

48. Refer to Figure 6.2. Identify the problem on the pressure–time graph of a COPD patient receiving CPAP + 5 cm $H_2O$ with pressure-support ventilation.

49. What can be done to correct the identified problem in Question 48?

_____

50. The flow cycling percentage is set to 20%, and the peak inspiratory flow is 50 L/min. At what flow rate will the ventilator cycle to exhalation?

_____

51. The flow cycling percentage is set to 40%, and the peak inspiratory flow is 50 L/min. At what flow rate will the ventilator cycle to exhalation?

52. Compare the answers for Questions 50 and 51. Which flow cycling set percentage will provide the shortest inspiratory time? Explain your answer.

53. What are the three ways of establishing the initial PIP during PCV?
    a. 
    b. 
    c. 

54. a. What are the initial setting ranges for BiPAP?

    b. What is the target tidal volume during BiPAP?

55. The ventilator mode where the breath is pressure limited, time cycled, and uses $V_T$ as a feedback control is _____.

56. How does the Servo-i establish initial pressure in the PRVC mode?

57. Why is it important to set an upper pressure limit during PRVC?

58. During ventilation of a patient with PRVC, the respiratory therapist notes that there is an audible alarm and a digital message that says "pressure limit, please evaluate." List four causes of this problem.

59. Explain how $P_{alv}$ is estimated during PC-CMV.

## CRITICAL THINKING QUESTIONS

1. What considerations need to be made by the respiratory therapist before initiating mechanical ventilation?

2. How do changes in the compliance affect the airway pressure and exhaled tidal volume in the volume-controlled mode compared to the pressure-control mode?

3. What two safety systems do ventilators have to end inspiration during PSV?

## CASE STUDIES

*Case Study*

A 28-year-old woman presents to the emergency department with complaints of difficulty breathing, general muscle weakness, and dysphagia. Her history of present illness reveals that she was diagnosed with infectious mononucleosis 10 days ago and has recently experienced ptosis and weakness in her legs and arms. She weighs 150 pounds and is 5 feet 8 inches tall. Arterial blood gas analysis on room air reveals pH 7.30, $P_aCO_2$ 50 mm Hg, $PO_2$ 78 mm Hg, $S_aO_2$ 91%, and $HCO_3^-$ 23 mEq/L. Her maximal inspiratory pressure is 15 cm $H_2O$ and VC is 13 mL/kg.

1. What is the most appropriate action at this time?

2. Calculate the patient's minute ventilation using the Dubois Body Surface Chart in Figure 6.1.

3. What tidal volume and respiratory rate ranges would be appropriate for this patient?

_____

Fifteen minutes later, the patient's breathing is very shallow; she is unresponsive and is immediately intubated.

4. Suggest an appropriate mode of ventilation for this patient? Explain your choice.

_____

5. What ventilator settings would you recommend?

_____

## NBRC-STYLE QUESTIONS

1. A 6-foot-tall male patient with pulmonary fibrosis is being ventilated in VC-CMV, rate 10 breaths/min, $V_T$ 600 mL, $F_IO_2$ 0.50, and PEEP +10 cm $H_2O$. The patient's PIP is 53 cm $H_2O$, and the $P_{plateau}$ is 47 cm $H_2O$. It is decided to switch the patient to PC-CMV. What set PIP will deliver 6 mL/kg IBW?
   a. 30 cm $H_2O$
   b. 35 cm $H_2O$
   c. 38 cm $H_2O$
   d. 43 cm $H_2O$

2. The most appropriate initial settings for a 5-foot 4-inch-tall female postoperative patient with no lung disease would be which of the following?
   a. PC-CMV, PIP 35 cm $H_2O$, f 20 breaths/min, PEEP +10 cm $H_2O$
   b. PC-SIMV, PIP 20 cm $H_2O$, f 6 breaths/min, PEEP +8 cm $H_2O$
   c. VC-CMV, 450 mL, f 10 breaths/min, PEEP +5 cm $H_2O$
   d. VC-CMV, 700 mL, f 14 breaths/min, PEEP 0 cm $H_2O$

3. A patient is ready to be changed from VC-IMV to PSV. The VC-IMV settings were $V_T$ 450 mL, f 4 breaths/min, and PEEP +5 cm $H_2O$. The patient's PIP is 31 cm $H_2O$, and $P_{plateau}$ is 23 cm $H_2O$. The initial PSV setting for this patient should be which of the following?
   a. 5 cm $H_2O$
   b. 8 cm $H_2O$
   c. 10 cm $H_2O$
   d. 12 cm $H_2O$

4. The flow waveform that is most appropriate for a patient with a high $R_{aw}$ is which of the following?
   a. Rectangle
   b. Descending
   c. Ascending
   d. Exponential

5. Calculate the I:E ratio when the set rate is 35 breaths/min and the $T_I$ = 1 second.
   a. 1:1
   b. 1.4:1
   c. 1.7:1
   d. 2:1

6. What flow rate is necessary to deliver a $V_T$ of 500 mL at a rate of 15 breaths/min with an I:E ratio of 1:3?
   a. 30 L/min
   b. 35 L/min
   c. 40 L/min
   d. 45 L/min

7. The appropriate minute ventilation for a male with a BSA of 2.3 $m^2$ and a body temperature of 40°C is which of the following?
   a. 8.2 L/min
   b. 9.6 L/min
   c. 10.6 L/min
   d. 11.7 L/min

8. A 5-foot 1-inch-tall female patient receiving PSV 6 cm $H_2O$ is showing signs of accessory muscle use and is exhaling a $V_T$ of 220 mL at a rate of 28 breaths/min. The most appropriate action at this time is which of the following?
   a. Adjust the $FIO_2$.
   b. Increase the set flow rate.
   c. Increase the PSV to 10 cm $H_2O$.
   d. Adjust the flow cycling percentage.

9. A 5-foot 7-inch-tall female multiple trauma patient was being managed on VC-CMV, f 12 breaths/min, $V_T$ 640 mL, PEEP +5 cm $H_2O$, $F_IO_2$ 60%, and a constant waveform for the past 24 hours. Currently, PIP is 45 cm $H_2O$, $P_{plateau}$ is 38 cm $H_2O$, and the patient has been diagnosed with acute respiratory distress syndrome. The respiratory therapist wants to switch the patient to PC-CMV. The initial pressure setting to target the appropriate $V_T$ for this patient is which of the following?
   a. 10 cm $H_2O$
   b. 20 cm $H_2O$
   c. 38 cm $H_2O$
   d. 45 cm $H_2O$

10. How is pressure-support ventilation cycled?
    a. Flow
    b. Pressure
    c. Volume
    d. Time

# 7 Final Considerations in Ventilator Setup

## LEARNING OBJECTIVES

*Upon completion of this chapter, the reader will be able to do the following:*

1. Recommend fractional inspired oxygen concentration ($F_IO_2$) settings when initiating mechanical ventilation.
2. Discuss the pros and cons of using the sigh function during mechanical ventilation.
3. Compare the use of sigh with the concept of a recruitment maneuver in acute respiratory distress syndrome.
4. List the actions necessary for final ventilator setup.
5. Explain the concept of using extrinsic positive end-expiratory pressure in patients with airflow obstruction and air trapping who have trouble triggering a breath during mechanical ventilation.
6. Calculate the desired $F_IO_2$ setting given the current partial pressure of arterial oxygen ($P_aO_2$) and $F_IO_2$ values.
7. List the essential capabilities of an adult intensive care unit ventilator.
8. Provide initial ventilator settings from the guidelines for patient management for any of the following patient conditions: chronic obstructive pulmonary disease, acute asthma exacerbation, neuromuscular disorders, closed head injuries, acute respiratory distress syndrome, and acute cardiogenic pulmonary edema.

**KEY TERMS CROSSWORD PUZZLE**

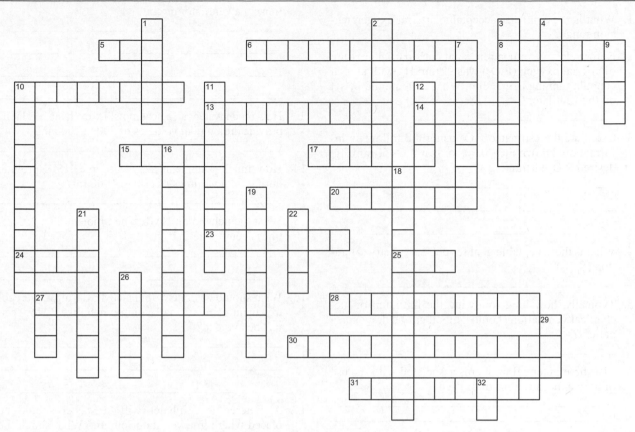

## Across

5 A type of pressure measured to determine brain swelling in a patient with a closed head injury (abbreviation)
6 Pharmacologic agent that can improve myocardial oxygenation and reduce preload and afterload
8 The typical color of sputum in the presence of respiratory infection
10 The sound sometimes associated with alveoli popping open during inspiration
13 A pharmacologic agent given to improve cardiac contractility
14 Warn of possible dangers
15 Too much air in the lungs causes this type of resonance
17 The preferred method of patient trigger that has a rapid response time
20 Type of water with which a humidifier is filled
23 The normal response to acute increases in intracranial pressure (ICP)
24 A chemical administered to keep pH in an acceptable range (abbreviation)
25 The pressure required to maintain cerebral blood flow (abbreviation)
27 The process of adding fluids
28 Excess pressure in the lungs can cause this
30 Not in sync
31 Low amount of oxygen in the blood

## Down

1 Type of alarm that warns when the patient stops breathing
2 Type of score used to evaluate a patient's neurologic responses
3 Type of hyperinflation that occurs with auto-PEEP
4 The neuromuscular disease that was made famous by a ball player (abbreviation)
7 A percentage of absolute humidity compared with capacity
9 A humidifier that uses the capillary action
10 Presence of this in the circuit tubing can potentially be a source of accidental lavage
11 Type of medications given to reduce vascular fluid load
12 Interface for noninvasive ventilation
16 Knowingly allowing the carbon dioxide levels to rise during mechanical ventilation is known as _____ hypercapnia.
18 A look-and-see type of pulmonary diagnostic procedure
19 One type of humidifier
21 Type of deficit that increases when dry gas is inhaled
22 This type of breath is used for lung recruitment
26 Type of alarm that warns when the inspiratory time exceeds the expiratory time
27 An artificial nose (abbreviation)
29 The point at which inhaled air reaches 100% relative humidity (abbreviation)
32 A neuromuscular disease with rapid onset (abbreviation)

## CHAPTER REVIEW QUESTIONS

1. What is the clinically acceptable arterial oxygen tension range?

2. Before elective intubation, a patient's partial pressure of arterial oxygen ($P_aO_2$) was 92 mm Hg with a nasal cannula running at 2 L/min. What $F_IO_2$ should be set on the ventilator?

   _____

3. Calculate the estimated $F_IO_2$ using the following information: known $F_IO_2$ 0.50, known $P_aO_2$ 60 mm Hg, desired $P_aO_2$ 90 mm Hg.

   _____

   _____

   _____

4. What is the acceptable goal for pulse oximetry saturation ($S_pO_2$)?

   _____

5. Typically, how long following the initiation of mechanical ventilation should a blood gas be drawn on a patient?

   _____

6. List three potential problems associated with the use of high concentrations of oxygen.
   a. _____
   b. _____
   c. _____

7. Why does flow triggering have a faster response time than pressure triggering?

   _____

   _____

   _____

8. Explain how auto-PEEP may interfere with pressure triggering?

   _____

   _____

   _____

9. What is the isothermic saturation boundary? Where is it located?

   _____

10. What should the absolute humidity of a ventilator's humidification system be? What temperatures should it be between?

    _____

    _____

11. List two advantages of a closed humidification system.
    a. _____
    b. _____

12. Explain what causes excessive rain-out (condensation) in a ventilator circuit.

    _____

    _____

    _____

    _____

13. How much water can a heat moisture exchanger (HME) provide during tidal volumes of 500 to 1000 mL?

    _____

14. How much water can a hygroscopic HME provide during tidal volumes of 500 to 1000 mL?

    _____

15. What happens to an HME when moisture and secretions accumulate in it?

    _____

    _____

16. What should be done with the HME during an aerosol treatment using a small-volume nebulizer? How can this be avoided?

    _____

    _____

    _____

17. A metered-dose inhaler with a spacer should be placed where in a ventilator circuit? What should be done with the HME?

    _____

    _____

    _____

18. List five contraindications to the use of HMEs.
    a. _____
    b. _____
    c. _____
    d. _____
    e. _____

19. List and explain the three levels of alarms that can happen during mechanical ventilation.
    a. _____
    b. _____
    c. _____

For Questions 20 through 35, identify the alarm situations with the appropriate alarm level.
**Select 1, 2, or 3**.

20. _____ Heater/humidifier malfunction

21. _____ Timing failure

22. _____ Autocycling

23. _____ Auto-PEEP

24. _____ Excessive gas delivery to the patient

25. _____ Inappropriate PEEP/continuous positive airway pressure (CPAP)

26. _____ Exhalation valve failure

27. _____ Inspiratory-to-expiratory ratio (I:E ratio) inappropriate

28. _____ Electrical power failure

29. _____ Changes in lung characteristics

30. _____ Circuit leak

31. _____ No gas delivery to the patient

32. _____ Electrical power failure

33. _____ Circuit partially obstructed

34. _____ Inappropriate oxygen level

35. _____ Changes in ventilatory drive

36. Following the application of VC- continuous mandatory ventilation (CMV) with +8 cm $H_2O$ PEEP to a patient, the respiratory therapist notices that the average peak inspiratory pressure (PIP) is 30 cm $H_2O$. What values would you suggest for the low-pressure, high-pressure, and low PEEP alarms to be set?
_____

37. The maximum value at which the apnea alarm should be set with any ventilator is how many seconds?
_____

38. Describe the similarity between lung recruitment strategies and sigh maneuvers.
_____
_____
_____

39. List four circumstances where sighs or deep breaths are appropriate.
   a. _____
   b. _____
   c. _____
   d. _____

40. List the ten steps the respiratory therapist should perform on the ventilator and other related equipment during the final preparation of ventilator set up.
   a. _____
   b. _____
   c. _____
   d. _____
   e. _____
   f. _____
   g. _____
   h. _____
   i. _____
   j. _____

41. Once the decision has been made to place a patient on mechanical ventilation, what steps should the respiratory therapist take?
   a. _____
   b. _____
   c. _____
   d. _____
   e. _____
   f. _____

42. List the essential capabilities of an adult ventilator.
   a. Mode: _____
   b. Tidal volume range: _____
   c. Respiratory rate range: _____
   d. Pressure range: _____
   e. PEEP/CPAP range: _____
   f. Flow rate range: _____
   g. Flow waveform: _____
   h. $F_IO_2$: _____
   i. Diagnostic measurement: _____
   j. Alarm: _____

43. What lung characteristics do patients with COPD typically exhibit?
_____

44. What is the primary reason for mechanical ventilator support for patients with COPD?
_____

45. List five causes of increased morbidity for COPD patients receiving mechanical ventilation.
   a. _____
   b. _____
   c. _____
   d. _____
   e. _____

46. The guidelines for mechanical ventilation of COPD patients suggest which mode of choice, if possible?
_____

47. The intubation route of choice as suggested by the guidelines for a patient with COPD is
_____.

48. Complete the following chart summarizing the ventilator guidelines for COPD patients.

| Parameter | Preferred Setting or Range |
|---|---|
| Tidal volume | _____ |
| Rate | _____ |
| Inspiratory time | _____ |
| Flow rate | _____ |
| Flow waveform | _____ |
| PEEP | _____ |
| $F_IO_2$ | _____ |

49. Define *pulsus paradoxus*.
_____
_____
_____

50. What are the two main concerns that a respiratory therapist must be aware of during the mechanical ventilation of a patient with acute asthma?
   a. _____
   b. _____

51. Where should the plateau pressure be kept during ventilation of a patient with asthma?

52. Complete the following chart summarizing the ventilator guidelines for patients with acute severe asthma.

| Parameter | Preferred Setting or Range |
|---|---|
| Tidal volume | _____ |
| Rate | _____ |
| Inspiratory time | _____ |
| Flow rate | _____ |
| Flow waveform | _____ |
| PEEP | _____ |
| $F_IO_2$ | _____ |

53. What is typically revealed during diagnostic percussion during an asthma episode?
_____

54. List five neuromuscular disorders that may require ventilatory support.
   a. _____
   b. _____
   c. _____
   d. _____
   e. _____

55. What are the main reasons that patients with neuromuscular disorders may require ventilatory support?
_____
_____

56. Complete the following chart summarizing the ventilator guidelines for patients with neuromuscular disorders.

| Parameter | Preferred Setting or Range |
|---|---|
| Tidal volume | _____ |
| Rate | _____ |
| Inspiratory time | _____ |
| Flow rate | _____ |
| Flow waveform | _____ |
| PEEP | _____ |
| $F_IO_2$ | _____ |

57. What are the common causes of increased ICPs?
_____
_____
_____

58. As it relates to cerebral perfusion pressure (CPP):
   a. What is the equation for CPP?
   _____

   b. What are the normal values for the components of this formula?
   _____

59. What CPP indicates poor cerebral perfusion?
_____

60. When and how should iatrogenic hyperventilation be used?
_____

61. Complete the following chart summarizing the ventilator guidelines for patients with closed head injury.

| Parameter | Preferred Setting or Range |
|---|---|
| Tidal volume | _____ |
| Rate | _____ |
| Inspiratory time | _____ |
| Flow rate | _____ |
| Flow waveform | _____ |
| PEEP | _____ |
| $F_IO_2$ | _____ |

62. List the diagnostic criteria for ARDS.
   a. _____
   b. _____
   c. _____
   d. _____
   e. _____

63. List ten examples of conditions associated with the development of ARDS.
   a. _____
   b. _____
   c. _____
   d. _____
   e. _____
   f. _____
   g. _____
   h. _____
   i. _____
   j. _____

64. Describe the open lung approach to ventilating patients with ARDS.
_____
_____
_____

65. Complete the following chart summarizing the ventilator guidelines for patients with ARDS.

| Parameter | Preferred Setting or Range |
| --- | --- |
| Tidal volume | _____ |
| Rate | _____ |
| Inspiratory time | _____ |
| Flow rate | _____ |
| Flow waveform | _____ |
| PEEP | _____ |
| $F_IO_2$ | _____ |

66. In the management of ARDS, what are the acceptable end points for arterial blood gases?

_____

_____

67. How is refractory hypoxemia identified?

_____

68. How does ARDS present on chest x-ray?

_____

69. What total lung compliance with a patient with ARDS typically have?

_____

_____

70. What is the amount of pulmonary shunt that is indicative of ARDS?

_____

_____

71. What is the pulmonary capillary wedge pressure values that are typically found in patients with ARDS?

_____

_____

72. Five common causes of acute cardiogenic pulmonary edema and congestive heart failure (CHF) include:
    a. _____
    b. _____
    c. _____
    d. _____
    e. _____

73. Complete the following chart summarizing the ventilator guidelines for patients with CHF.

| Parameter | Preferred Setting or Range |
| --- | --- |
| Tidal volume | _____ |
| Rate | _____ |
| Inspiratory time | _____ |
| Flow rate | _____ |
| Flow waveform | _____ |
| PEEP | _____ |
| $F_IO_2$ | _____ |

74. Patients with CHF and mild to moderate hypoxemia can be successfully managed without intubation using which two modalities?

_____

_____

## CRITICAL THINKING QUESTIONS

1. Discuss the pros and cons of using sighs with mechanical ventilation.

_____

_____

_____

_____

_____

2. Explain the progression of an asthma episode from arrival at the emergency department to intubation and mechanical ventilation.

_____

_____

_____

_____

_____

_____

_____

3. Discuss why the use of pressure-support ventilation (PSV) may not be appropriate for patients with COPD.

_____

_____

_____

_____

_____

_____

4. Why is it important for expiratory time to be maximized when ventilating a patient with increased airway resistance, such as with asthma or COPD?

_____

_____

_____

## CASE STUDIES

### Case Study 1

A 62-year-old male weighs 256 pounds and is 73 inches tall. The patient has a history of congestive heart failure and has been placed on a nonrebreathing mask at 15 L/min. Physical assessment reveals that the patient is alert and oriented but anxious and diaphoretic. Vital signs are as follows: pulse 142 beats/min and thready, blood pressure 105/68 mm Hg, oral temperature 98.6° F, and respiratory rate 26 breaths/min, shallow and labored. Breath sounds reveal bilateral inspiratory coarse crackles. The arterial blood gas on the nonrebreathing mask is pH 7.24, $P_aCO_2$ 51 mm Hg, $P_aO_2$ 42 mm Hg, and $HCO_3^-$ 23 mEq/L. The patient's electrocardiogram shows a widened QRS complex with occasional premature ventricular contractions.

1. What respiratory care intervention is indicated at this time?

   _____

   _____

2. If this patient is intubated and placed on mechanical ventilation, what mode, tidal volume, and rate would you suggest?

   _____

   _____

### Case Study 2

A motor vehicle crash victim arrives at the hospital via ambulance. The 37-year-old woman has sustained a closed head injury. Physical assessment reveals a pulse of 145 beats/min, respiratory rate 32 breaths/min, and blood pressure 155/97 mm Hg. Her neck veins are distended, and she is diaphoretic. She is 68 inches tall and weighs 175 pounds. The patient has no history of cardiac or respiratory disease. The patient has an oral airway in place with a weak gag reflex. On 60% oxygen, the arterial blood gas is pH 7.22, $P_aCO_2$ 64 mm Hg, $P_aO_2$ 78 mm Hg, $S_aO_2$ 92%, and $HCO_3^-$ 25 mEq/L.

1. What type of respiratory failure appears to be present in this patient?

   _____

   _____

2. What acid–base imbalance is present?

   _____

3. What type of mechanical ventilatory support may this patient benefit from?

   _____

4. What are the appropriate parameters for this patient, including minute ventilation, tidal volume, inspiratory time, flow rate, and PEEP?

   _____

   _____

## Case Study 3

A 40-year-old female, height 66 inches and weight 156 pounds, presents to the emergency department with the chief complaint of shortness of breath. She is alert, very anxious, unable to complete a sentence without stopping to take a breath, and is sitting in a tripod position. Her heart rate is 136 beats/min and regular; respirations are 30 breaths/min and very labored with accessory muscle use. Her blood pressure is 168/84 mm Hg, and her oral temperature is 37.2° C. Breath sounds are decreased bilaterally with expiratory wheezes. She has a weak, nonproductive cough. The patient has been receiving continuous aerosol albuterol and has received intravenous Solu-Medrol. The patient's best peak flow after bronchodilator therapy is 150 L/min, with her normal best typically around 500 L/min. Arterial blood gas results while on a nasal cannula at 6 L/min show pH 7.34, $P_aCO_2$ 42 mm Hg, $P_aO_2$ 48 mm Hg, $S_aO_2$ 79%, and $HCO_3^-$ 22 mEq/L.

1. How should this blood gas be interpreted?

2. Does the situation warrant intubation and mechanical ventilation? Why or why not?

3. What type of mechanical ventilatory support may this patient benefit from?

4. If pressure-controlled (PC)-CMV is used for this patient, what are the appropriate settings (including PIP setting, resulting tidal volume, respiratory rate, inspiratory time, waveform, and PEEP)?

## Case Study 4

A 64-year-old, 197-pound, 6-foot 1-inch male patient was admitted 3 days ago for a COPD exacerbation. He is currently receiving supplemental oxygen via nasal cannula at 3 L/min, albuterol and ipratropium every 4 hours, and an intravenous corticosteroid and antibiotic. He has bilaterally diminished breath sounds, with rhonchi in both bases and a weak, nonproductive cough. A chest x-ray from this morning shows bibasilar infiltrates. The current arterial blood gas results reveal pH 7.32, $P_aCO_2$ 57 mm Hg, $P_aO_2$ 54 mm Hg, $S_aO_2$ 85%, and $HCO_3^-$ 29 mEq/L.

1. How should this blood gas be interpreted?

2. Does the situation warrant intubation and mechanical ventilation? Why or why not?

3. If intubation is required, what mode and parameters would you suggest for this patient?

## NBRC-STYLE QUESTIONS

1. Which of the following are true concerning the use of permissive hypercapnia in the management of ARDS?
    1. Keep $P_{plat}$ below 30 cm $H_2O$ by lowering the $V_T$ to 4 to 6 mL/kg.
    2. $P_aCO_2$ should go no higher than 60 mm Hg.
    3. High $PEEP_E$ levels greater than 15 cm $H_2O$ may be required.
    4. The $P_aCO_2$ is permitted to rise rapidly to the acceptable level.
    a. 1 and 3 only
    b. 2 and 4 only
    c. 1 and 4 only
    d. 2 and 3 only

2. A mechanically ventilated patient has been using an HME for humidification for the past 72 hours. During rounds and chart review, the respiratory therapist notices a steady increase in the PIP over the past 2 days. The respiratory therapist suctions the patient to assess the secretions. The secretions are very thick and tenacious. The most appropriate action at this time is which of the following?
    a. Suction the patient more often.
    b. Add a passover humidifier to the system.
    c. Switch to a heated wick-type humidifier.
    d. Use normal saline to lavage before suctioning.

3. A 75-year-old woman, admitted through the emergency department earlier today, is increasingly distressed and unable to breathe comfortably except in the upright position. She has a history of coronary artery disease, and on admission, she was complaining of chest pain. She is becoming increasingly short of breath and appears cyanotic. Vital signs reveal pulse 142 beats/min, blood pressure 150/92 mm Hg, and respiratory rate 30 breaths/min and labored. The arterial blood gas on nasal cannula 3 L/min is pH 7.18, $P_aCO_2$ 81 mm Hg, $P_aO_2$ 35 mm Hg, $S_aO_2$ 79%, and $HCO_3^-$ 29 mEq/L. The respiratory therapist should recommend which of the following?
    a. Nasal mask CPAP at +10 cm $H_2O$
    b. Nonrebreathing mask with 15 L/min oxygen
    c. Bilevel PAP: inspiratory positive airway pressure (IPAP) 15 cm $H_2O$ and expiratory positive airway pressure (EPAP) 5 cm $H_2O$
    d. Intubation and mechanical ventilation with PCCMV

4. Appropriate ventilatory parameters for an otherwise healthy 185-pound, 6-foot 1-inch, 26-year-old man who was brought to the emergency department because of a drug overdose include which of the following?
    a. VC-CMV, tidal volume 600 mL, set rate 12 breaths/min
    b. VC-IMV, tidal volume 600 mL, set rate 6 breaths/min
    c. PC-CMV, set pressure 25 cm $H_2O$, inspiratory time 1.5 seconds
    d. Pressure support ventilation of 15 cm $H_2O$ with CPAP 5 cm $H_2O$

5. Before intubation, a patient's $P_aO_2$ was 78 mm Hg while receiving an $F_IO_2$ of 0.60. What $F_IO_2$ setting on the ventilator will bring the $P_aO_2$ up to 90 mm Hg? (Assume that this patient's cardiopulmonary status and respiratory quotient are constant.)
    a. 0.70
    b. 0.75
    c. 0.80
    d. 0.85

6. A 64-year-old obese man with suspected drug overdose has just been intubated in the emergency department. The patient is 6 feet tall and weighs 435 pounds. The most appropriate tidal volume to ventilate this patient is which of the following?
    a. 380 mL
    b. 640 mL
    c. 810 mL
    d. 975 mL

7. Which of the following ventilatory parameters is appropriate when mechanically ventilating a patient with COPD?
    a. Use a rectangle flow waveform.
    b. Set the tidal volume between 10 and 15 mL/kg.
    c. Use peak inspiratory flow rates greater than 60 L/min.
    d. Institute PEEP in the range of 5 to 10 cm $H_2O$.

8. A patient with ARDS has been changed from VCCMV to PC-CMV. When this change was made, there was an increase in the mean airway pressure. Which of the following statements is true concerning elevated mean airway pressures?
    a. The mean airway pressure increases with longer expiratory times.
    b. An increased mean airway pressure may result in improved oxygenation.
    c. Elevated mean airway pressures decrease the risk of barotrauma.
    d. High mean airway pressures increase the risk of cardiovascular side effects.

9. A 5-feet 4-inch-tall, 125-pound woman who has just been intubated because of a severe asthma episode would be ventilated most appropriately with which of the following ventilator parameters?
    a. PSV 20 cm $H_2O$ with CPAP +10 cm $H_2O$
    b. PC-CMV, 12 breath/min, PIP 25 cm $H_2O$, $T_I$ 0.75 second
    c. VC-IMV, 12 breath/min, $V_T$ 800 mL, flow 50 L/min, rectangle waveform
    d. VC-CMV, 10 breath/min, $V_T$ 570 mL, flow 35 L/min, descending waveform

10. HMEs may not be appropriate for use with infants, children, and small adults due to which of the following?
    a. Presence of mechanical dead space in the HMEs
    b. Increased rate of endotracheal occlusion with these patients
    c. Patients' inability to overcome resistance across the HME
    d. HME's inability to provide adequate humidity for these patients

# 8 | Initial Patient Assessment

## LEARNING OBJECTIVES

*Upon completion of this chapter, the reader will be able to do the following:*

1. Understand the importance of performing an operational verification procedure.
2. State the recommended times when an oxygen analyzer is used to measure the fractional inspired oxygen concentration ($F_IO_2$) during mechanical ventilation.
3. Identify various pathophysiological conditions that alter a patient's transairway pressure, peak pressure, and plateau pressure.
4. Use pressure–time and flow–time curves obtained during pressure-controlled continuous mandatory ventilation to determine the plateau pressure.
5. Identify a system leak from a volume–time curve.
6. Use physical examination and radiographic data to determine whether pneumonia, acute respiratory distress syndrome, flail chest, pneumothorax, asthma, pleural effusion, or emphysema is present.
7. Determine whether a lung compliance problem or an airway resistance problem is present, using the ventilator flow sheet and time, volume, peak inspiratory pressure, and plateau pressure data.
8. Evaluate a static pressure–volume curve for static compliance and dynamic compliance to determine changes in compliance or resistance.
9. Estimate a patient's alveolar ventilation based on the ideal body weight, tidal volume, and respiratory rate.
10. Detect a cuff leak by listening to breath sounds.
11. Recognize inappropriate endotracheal tube cuff pressures and an inappropriate tube size and recommend measures to correct these problems.
12. Evaluate flow sheet information about a patient on pressure control ventilation and recommend methods for determining whether compliance and airway resistance have changed.
13. Explain the technique for measuring endotracheal tube cuff pressure using a manometer, syringe, and three-way stopcock.
14. Describe two methods that can be used to remedy a cut pilot tube (pilot balloon line) without changing the endotracheal tube.

## KEY TERMS CROSSWORD PUZZLE

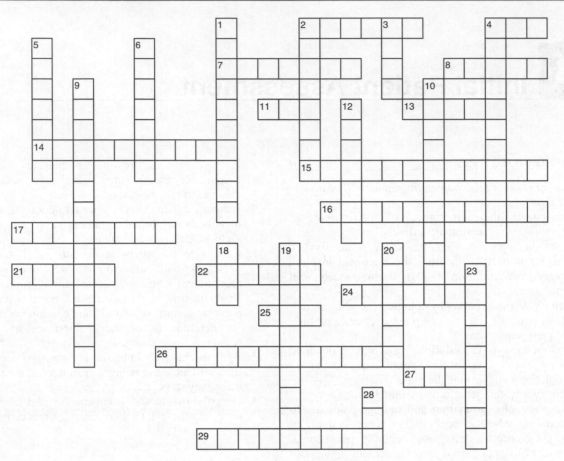

### Across

2 A place to measure temperature
4 Something in the ventilator circuit that adds dead space (abbreviation)
7 A cause of abdominal distention due to fluid
8 The _____ inflection point indicates a time at which large numbers of alveoli are becoming overinflated.
11 A multipart procedure to check that a ventilator is working properly (abbreviation)
13 A cuffed endotracheal tube has a _____ balloon.
14 A common place for leaks
15 It puts air in the pleural space and reduces lung compliance
16 The setting that allows patient triggering
17 Cell death
21 The _____ inflection point indicates the pressure at which large numbers of alveoli are being recruited.
22 Type of compliance measured at no flow
24 Type of compliance that is measured during gas movement
25 A pressure that can be measured continuously by a flow-directed catheter (abbreviation)
26 Another term used to describe tubing compliance is _____ volume.
27 Another name for base flow is _____ flow.
29 The form on which the patient–ventilator check is written (two words)

### Down

1 Type of pressure that is important to tissue oxygenation and affects both lung volumes and cardiac output (two words)
2 Dynamic hyperinflation (two words)
3 When the exhaled tidal volume is less than the set tidal volume, there is a _____.
4 A condition of low body temperature
5 A breath sound that indicates the possible need for suctioning
6 A type of recoil
9 It puts fluid in the alveoli and reduces lung compliance (two words)
10 A place where the central venous pressure catheter dwells (two words)
12 A breath sound that indicates the possible need for bronchodilator therapy
18 The amount of pressure needed to overcome airway resistance (abbreviation)
19 Heart rate, respiratory rate, and blood pressure are all part of this (two words)
20 Tidal volume multiplied by respiratory rate (frequency) equals _____ ventilation
23 The secondary respiratory muscles
28 Method for ensuring no leaks around an endotracheal tube (abbreviation)

## CHAPTER REVIEW QUESTIONS

1. List eight observations that the clinician should make when assessing the physiologic status of a patient receiving mechanical ventilation.

   a. _____

   b. _____

   c. _____

   d. _____

   e. _____

   f. _____

   g. _____

   h. _____

2. Typically, where is the documentation of patient information and ventilator settings made?

3. Before a ventilator can be used on a patient, the respiratory therapist must confirm this procedure was performed and passed on that ventilator.

   _____

4. In addition to regularly timed checks, list six instances when patient–ventilator system checks should be performed.

   a. _____

   b. _____

   c. _____

   d. _____

   e. _____

   f. _____

5. If continuous $F_IO_2$ measurement is not available on a particular ventilator, how often should it be measured for:

   a. An adult?

   b. An infant?

6. What is the first thing the clinician should assess following a patient being connected to a mechanical ventilator?

   _____

7. How long should a clinician wait after the initiation of mechanical ventilation to draw an arterial blood gas sample?

   _____

8. What is an appropriate range for pressure-trigger setting (sensitivity setting)?

   _____

9. What is an appropriate range for flow triggering setting (sensitivity setting)?

10. a. How does auto-PEEP (positive end-expiratory pressure) make triggering the ventilator more difficult for a patient?

    b. How can triggering the ventilator be made easier without causing autotriggering?

    a. _____

    b. _____

11. Describe a strategy that may be used to eliminate or reduce auto-PEEP.

    _____

    _____

    _____

    _____

12. What effect would a heat moisture exchanger attached to the endotracheal tube have on alveolar ventilation?

    _____

    _____

13. Calculate the alveolar minute ventilation if the set $V_T$ is 775 mL, ideal body weight is 160 pounds, and added $V_D$ is 85 mL.

    _____

    _____

14. List two factors to consider when determining alveolar ventilation.

    a. _____

    b. _____

15. What changes in compliance or airway resistance can cause an increase in PIP?

    _____

16. What ventilator maneuver must be performed to measure the plateau pressure?

    _____

17. Describe a clinical scenario that would result in an inaccurate plateau pressure measurement.

    _____

    _____

18. Ideally, to avoid lung injury, at what level or below, should a plateau pressure be kept?

19. What pressure measurements are needed to calculate dynamic compliance?

    _____

20. What pressure measurements are needed to calculate static compliance?

    _____

21. Define *transairway pressure*.

    _____

    _____

22. What does an increase in the difference between PIP and P$_{plat}$ indicate?

_____

_____

23. List four possible causes for increased airway resistance in a patient on mechanical ventilation.

    a. _____

    b. _____

    c. _____

    d. _____

24. What is the significance of monitoring mean airway pressure?

_____

_____

25. What maneuver is performed to assess auto-PEEP?

_____

26. What is a high pressure limit alarm usually set at? What happens when it is activated?

_____

27. List four possible causes that would activate the high pressure limit alarm.

    a. _____

    b. _____

    c. _____

    d. _____

28. What is the low pressure alarm is usually set at? What does it mean when it is activated?

_____

29. What is a common cause of activation of the low pressure alarm?

_____

30. If the leak is not obvious, what should you do while you further investigate the source?

_____

31. What are two methods the clinician can use to determine whether a leak is present?

    a. _____

    b. _____

32. If a leak is present, what steps should be taken to find the source?

_____

_____

_____

33. What effect would a leak have during pressure-support ventilation?

_____

34. Describe the following techniques used to inflate tube cuffs:

    a. Minimum occlusion technique:

    _____

    b. Minimum leak technique:

    _____

35. List the factors that can cause hyperthermia.

_____

_____

_____

36. The central venous pressure (CVP) directly reflects what pressures?

_____

_____

37. At what point during a ventilator breath should the CVP measurement be taken?

_____

38. Describe a clinical scenario where a patient would benefit from the monitoring of their pulmonary artery pressure.

_____

_____

39. How often should a physical examination of a ventilated patient be performed?

_____

40. What should be included in the physical examination?

_____

41. Describe the effect abdominal distention has on ventilation.

_____

42. Endotracheal or tracheostomy cuff pressure should be maintained in what range?

_____

43. Describe a clinical scenario where a cuff pressure of 25 mm Hg could cause tracheal damage.

_____

44. List the five-step protocol designed to minimize the risk of tracheal necrosis associated with endotracheal tube cuff overinflation.

    a. _____

    b. _____

    c. _____

    d. _____

    e. _____

45. List two situations in which a higher-than-acceptable cuff pressure may be required to maintain a minimal occlusion.

   a. _____

   b. _____

46. Describe the procedure for maintaining the cuff pressure if the pilot balloon is accidentally cut.

   _____

   _____

47. Why should an endotracheal tube be repositioned?

   _____

48. What is the normal value for static compliance ($C_S$)?

   _____

49. Writ the formula for $C_S$.

   _____

50. List eight possible causes for a decrease in $C_S$.

   a. _____

   b. _____

   c. _____

   d. _____

   e. _____

   f. _____

   g. _____

   h. _____

51. During pressure ventilation, if the set inspiratory pressure remains constant, what effect would a decreased $C_S$ have on the tidal volume ($V_T$)?

   _____

52. What is dynamic compliance ($C_D$)?

   _____

53. $C_D$ decreases whenever $C_S$ _____ or $R_{aw}$ _____.

54. During volume ventilation, what effect would a decrease in $C_D$ have on PIP and the delivered $V_T$?

   _____

   _____

55. Calculate the $C_S$ when the $V_T$ is 740 mL, $P_{plat}$ is 44 cm $H_2O$, and the end-expiratory pressure is +8 cm $H_2O$.

   _____

   _____

56. Calculate the $R_{aw}$ when the PIP is 58 cm $H_2O$, $P_{plat}$ is 51 cm $H_2O$, and the flow is 0.5 L/s.

   _____

   _____

   _____

57. Identify the problem in Figure 8.1.

   _____

58. What is the plateau pressure in Figure 8.2?

A    Time (seconds)

B    Time (seconds)

59. Calculate the static compliance for the information in Figure 8.2 using the returned tidal volume of 450 mL.

   _____

## CRITICAL THINKING QUESTIONS

1. During a patient–ventilator system check, the clinician notices the patient making inspiratory efforts (patient is using accessory muscles), but the ventilator is not triggering. What could be causing the problem? What steps could be taken to correct it?

   _____

   _____

   _____

   _____

2. A 250-pound adult man has a 6.5-mm inner diameter endotracheal tube in place and is being mechanically ventilated. Cuff pressures of 40 cm $H_2O$ are required to maintain an adequate seal. What recommendations should be made to correct this problem?

_____

_____

_____

_____

3. A patient with ARDS is being managed on pressure-controlled ventilation, with a set inspiratory pressure of 30 cm $H_2O$. According to the ventilator flow sheet, the measured tidal volumes for the past 3 days have ranged between 400 and 450 mL. During the first ventilator–patient system check of the day, the respiratory therapist notes that the measured tidal volume is now 550 mL, without any change in the set pressure parameters. What is likely the cause of the tidal volume increase?

_____

_____

_____

_____

4. When the PIP is 43 cm $H_2O$ and the plateau pressure is 18 cm $H_2O$, how much pressure is required to overcome the resistance of the airways?

_____

## CASE STUDIES

### Case Study 1

A respiratory therapist is called to a code in the intensive care unit (ICU). After the patient is stabilized, the physician writes the following order for mechanical ventilation: volume control, $V_T$ 700 mL, f 12, $F_IO_2$ 1.0, PEEP +5 cm $H_2O$. The respiratory therapist observes a PIP of 42 cm $H_2O$ with the order settings.

1. At what levels should the high- and low-pressure alarms be set?

_____

_____

2. At what level should the low $V_T$ alarm be set?

_____

3. How would the respiratory therapist obtain a plateau pressure?

_____

4. What should the therapist recommend if the plateau pressure measurement obtained was 38 cm $H_2O$?

_____

_____

_____

### Case Study 2

An obtunded patient in the ICU has been receiving volume ventilation CV-CMV for the past 3 days. Today the patient appears to be responsive and wakening up. The high-pressure, low-minute volume, and low tidal volume alarms are activating frequently, and the patient appears to be agitated and confused.

1. Indicate possible causes for the high-pressure alarm activating.

_____

_____

2. What could be a cause for the low-minute volume and low tidal volume alarms being activated?

_____

_____

3. What recommendations would you make to resolve the problem?

_____

_____

A 38-year-old female patient was admitted through the emergency department 24 hours ago following a motor vehicle crash. She was intubated in the field due to respiratory arrest secondary to blunt chest trauma. She also sustained four fractured ribs. The patient is currently on VC-CMV, f 15 breath/min, $V_T$ 440 mL, $F_IO_2$ 0.8, PEEP +8 cm $H_2O$. The following values were obtained on those ventilator settings.

| Time | PIP (cm $H_2O$) | $P_{plat}$ (cm $H_2O$) | Exhaled $V_T$ (mL) |
|------|------|------|------|
| 0800 | 35 | 30 | 440 |
| 1000 | 39 | 34 | 440 |
| 1100 | 45 | 39 | 440 |
| 1130 | 50 | 44 | 440 |

1. What is the $P_{ta}$ for each patient–ventilator system check?

_____

2. What is the likely cause for the increasing PIP over the course of the 3.5 hours?

_____

_____

_____

3. What are some of the most likely causes of this problem?

_____

_____

4. How would you assess the patient to determine the appropriate treatment?

_____

_____

_____

A 56-year-old male patient with a history of COPD was admitted yesterday with a diagnosis of pneumonia. During the night, he was intubated due to respiratory arrest. The patient is currently receiving VC-CMV, f 12 breath/min, $V_T$ 525 mL, $F_IO_2$ 0.4, and PEEP +3 cm $H_2O$. The following values were obtained on those ventilator settings.

| Time | PIP (cm $H_2O$) | $P_{plat}$ (cm $H_2O$) | Exhaled $V_T$ (mL) |
|------|------|------|------|
| 0630 | 36 | 23 | 525 |
| 0835 | 39 | 22 | 523 |
| 1030 | 41 | 23 | 525 |
| 1230 | 46 | 19 | 524 |

1. What is the $P_{ta}$ for each patient–ventilator system check?

_____

2. What is the likely cause for the increasing PIP over the course of the 6 hours?

_____

_____

_____

3. What are some of the most likely causes of this problem?

_____

_____

4. How would you assess and treat this patient?

_____

_____

_____

## NBRC-STYLE QUESTIONS

1. An increase in the peak inspiratory flow rate would increase which of the following?
   a. Tidal volume
   b. Total cycle time
   c. Expiratory time
   d. Inspiratory time

2. A patient receiving volume-controlled mechanical ventilation has a decrease in the static compliance. Which of the following would most likely occur?
   a. An increase in the tidal volume
   b. A decrease in the minute ventilation
   c. An increase in the PIP
   d. An increased inspiratory-to-expiratory ratio

3. While monitoring endotracheal cuff pressures during a patient-ventilator system check, the therapist obtains a reading of 44 cm $H_2O$. What should the therapist do next?
   a. Get a syringe and add air to the cuff.
   b. Insert a smaller diameter endotracheal tube.
   c. No changes need to be made; the cuff pressure is acceptable.
   d. Release air from the cuff until a minimal occluding volume is achieved.

4. Which of the following can cause a mechanically ventilated patient's PIP to increase from 20 to 40 cm $H_2O$ rapidly while the static compliance remains relatively unchanged?
   a. Recent removal of mucous plugs
   b. Decreased airway resistance
   c. Tension pneumothorax
   d. Decreased elastance

5. Which of the following can cause an increase in the PIP and plateau pressure with a stable transairway pressure?
   a. ARDS
   b. Acute asthma exacerbation
   c. Retained secretions in the airways
   d. An endotracheal tube that is too small

6. While responding to a ventilator alarm, the respiratory therapist sees that the low-pressure alarm is activated. She hears an audible leak, and notices that the exhaled volume is 200 mL below the set tidal volume. The measured cuff pressure is 15 mm Hg. What action should be taken next?
   a. Replace the endotracheal tube with a larger size.
   b. Increase the patient's $V_T$ to compensate for the leak.
   c. Introduce enough volume into the cuff to maintain a pressure of less than 20 cm $H_2O$.
   d. While auscultating the larynx, introduce enough air into the cuff until a slight leak is heard on peak inspiration.

7. Why is positive end-expiratory pressure (PEEP) subtracted from plateau pressure when calculating $C_s$?
   a. To compensate for a loss in volume due to a leak
   b. To determine auto-PEEP
   c. To determine the actual pressure change
   d. To calculate the actual PEEP level

8. Which of the following may cause an increase in heart rate?
   1. Hypoxemia
   2. Hypothermia
   3. Anxiety
   4. Pain
   a. 1 only
   b. 1 and 3 only
   c. 1, 2, and 3 only
   d. 1, 3, and 4 only

9. Which of the following physical findings would you expect when assessing an asthmatic patient?
   1. Late inspiratory crackles
   2. Hyper-resonant percussion note
   3. Accessory muscle use
   4. Tracheal shift
   a. 1 only
   b. 1 and 3 only
   c. 2 and 3 only
   d. 2, 3, and 4 only

10. Evaluate the following data from the patient's flow sheet.

| Time | Set $V_T$ | PIP (cm $H_2O$) | $P_{plat}$ (cm $H_2O$) |
|------|-----------|------------------|------------------------|
| 4:00 | 700 mL    | 38               | 32                     |
| 5:00 | 700 mL    | 41               | 34                     |
| 6:00 | 700 mL    | 47               | 32                     |

Based on the provided data, which of the following statements is true?
a. $C_L$ is improving.
b. There is no change in $C_L$.
c. $R_{aw}$ is improving.
d. There is an increase in $R_{aw}$.

# 9 Ventilator Graphics

## LEARNING OBJECTIVES

*On completion of this chapter, the reader will be able to do the following:*

1. Identify ventilator variables (e.g., the target variable and trigger variable) and ventilator parameters and their values (e.g., peak inspiratory pressure and plateau pressure) using pressure, flow, and volume scalars generated using various modes of mechanical ventilation.
2. Identify ventilator variables and ventilator parameters and their values from flow–volume and pressure–volume loops.
3. Use ventilator scalars and loops to detect changes in lung compliance and airway resistance, inappropriate sensitivity settings, inadequate inspiratory flow, auto-positive end-expiratory pressure (auto-PEEP), leaks in the ventilator circuit, active exhalation during pressure support ventilation, and an inspiratory pressure overshoot during pressure support ventilation.
4. Describe how changes in airway resistance and lung compliance affect scalars and loops during volume-targeted and pressure-targeted ventilation when airway resistance increases and lung compliances decreases.
5. Recognize periods of patient–ventilator asynchrony using scalars and loops.
6. Determine the presence of auto-PEEP using ventilator graphics.
7. Explain the phases of ventilation during airway pressure release ventilation using pressure and flow scalars.
8. Describe the relationship between airway and esophageal pressure changes using ventilator graphics.

**KEY TERMS CROSSWORD PUZZLE**

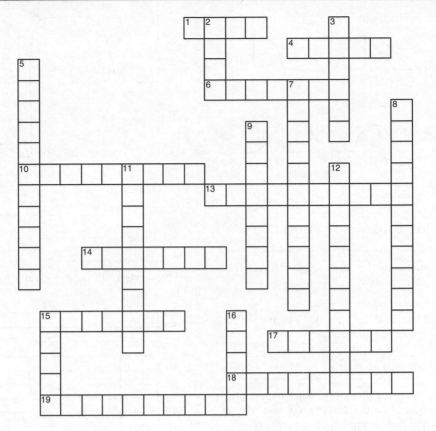

**Across**

1 Volume per unit of time
4 This control adjusts the rate at which the flow valve opens
6 Pressure reading when inspiration is held
10 Easy to inflate
13 The difference between the inspiratory and expiratory curves in a pressure–volume loop
14 Begins inspiration
15 A way to specify the waveforms for pressure, flow, and volume that are graphed against time
17 One variable plotted against time
18 Matching of the onset of breath by the ventilator and patient effort
19 The frictional forces associated with ventilation

**Down**

2 Two variables, other than time, plotted against each other
3 Flow multiplied by inspiratory time
5 When a patient and a ventilator are not working together
7 Rapid rise or decay on a graph
8 Name of pressure gradient required to overcome airway resistance
9 Type of flow that creates a wave form parallel to the *x*-axis
11 Type of positive end-expiratory pressure (PEEP) caused by air trapping
12 A square wave is also known as _____ .
15 Adjusting the rise of pressure or flow to the patient
16 This is necessary to measure plateau pressure

## CHAPTER REVIEW QUESTIONS

1. Identify the scalar shapes in Figure 9.1.

A. _____ B. _____ C. _____
D. _____ E. _____ F. _____

2. What is the difference between a scalar and a loop?

_____

3. What is the mathematical relationship between volume, flow, and inspiratory time?

_____

4. List the two factors that determine the flow of gas into the lungs.

a. _____

b. _____

5. As the lung compliance increases, what happens to the pressure required to deliver the volume to the patient? When the lung compliance decreases, what happens to the pressure required to deliver the volume to the patient?

_____

6. The pressure at the mouth ($P_{awo}$) is equal to the sum of what two pressures?

_____

7. When does the flow–time curve run parallel to the $x$-axis?

_____

8. Calculate the $T_I$ in seconds when the volume is 600 mL and the flow rate is 60 L/min.

_____

9. Calculate the $P_A$ when the delivered volume is 800 mL and static compliance is 25 mL/cm $H_2O$.

_____

10. Identify the labeled parts of the flow–time scalar in Figure 9.2.

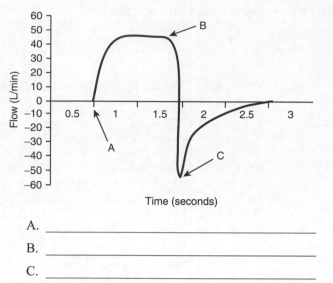

A. _____

B. _____

C. _____

For Questions 11 through 15, refer to the flow waveform in Figure 9.3.

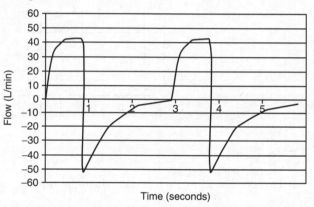

11. What type of flow waveform is shown in the figure?

_____

12. What is the peak inspiratory flow rate?

_____

13. What is the peak expiratory flow rate?

_____

14. What is the approximate inspiratory time?

_____

15. What is the expiratory time?

_____

16. You have a patient with an exacerbation of asthma, who was just intubated. The chest radiograph reveals a flattened diaphragm. What is the likely cause for the flow curve not returning to zero at the end of exhalation?

_____

17. Your patient was coughing when you attempted an inspiratory hold maneuver. Would the measurement be accurate? Why or why not?

_____

18. At what point in the breath cycle does the auto-PEEP measurement occur?

_____

19. In Figure 9.4, what is the reason for the increase in the flow (*point A*) at the end of inspiration?

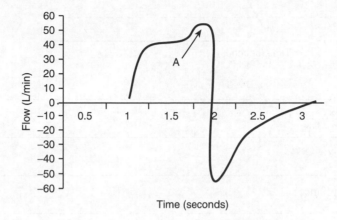

_____

20. What is the appropriate initial pressure trigger setting for an adult patient?

_____

21. Asynchrony between the patient and the ventilator may be caused by inappropriate settings of which two parameters?

_____

22. How does changing the flow pattern affect the PIP during volume ventilation?

_____

For Questions 23 through 29, refer to the pressure, volume, and flow curves for VC-CMV in the graphs in Figure 9.5.

23. What is the PIP?

_____

24. What is the set flow pattern and rate?

_____

25. What is the tidal volume?

_____

26. Calculate the static compliance.

_____

27. Calculate the airway resistance.

_____

28. Is intrinsic PEEP present? _____

29. Why does the flow rate drop to zero before the end of inspiration?

_____

30. During PCV, the patient's lung compliance drops. How will this affect the delivered volume?

_____

31. During PC-CMV, why does flow return to zero before the end of inspiration?

_____

32. What type of flow waveform is used during PCV?

_____

33. When does the highest pressure gradient between the ventilator and the lungs occur?

_____

34. What parameters need to be set to deliver PSV?

_____

35. Identify the ventilator mode from Figure 9.6.

For Questions 36 and 37, refer to Figure 9.7.

36. Identify the mode of ventilation.

_____

37. Identify waves *A* and *B*.

_____

38. Explain how automatic tube compensation works on inspiration and expiration.

_____

39. If the peak flow rate for a pressure support breath is 45 L/min and the flow cycle percent is set at 25%, at what flow rate will inspiration end?

_____

For Questions 40 through 44, refer to the flow curve for a PSV breath in Figure 9.8.

40. What is the $T_I$ for this breath?

_____

41. What is the peak inspiratory flow rate for this breath?

_____

42. At what flow rate did inspiration end?

_____

43. What is the flow cycle percent setting?

_____

44. What is the peak expiratory flow rate?

_____

45. Explain why a patient with chronic obstructive pulmonary disease (COPD) requires a higher flow cycle percent for PS breaths.

_____

46. Explain why a patient with stiff lungs gains the most benefit during PSV with a low flow cycle percent setting.

_____

For Questions 47 through 52, refer to the flow, pressure, and volume scalars represented in Figure 9.9. The scalars labeled *A* are the flow, pressure, and volume scalars for a single ventilator breath. The scalars labeled *B* refer to a second ventilator breath.

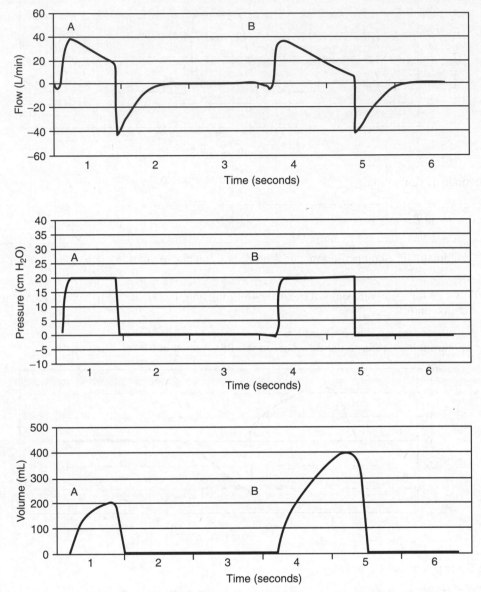

47. What is the approximate flow cycle percent in *A*?

_____

48. What is the patient tidal volume in *A*?

_____

49. What is the approximate flow cycle percent in *B*?

_____

50. What is the patient tidal volume in *B*?

_____

51. What are the approximate inspiratory times in breaths *A* and *B*?

_____

52. Why is the $T_I$ longer for *B* than for *A*?

_____

For Questions 53 through 56, refer to the pressure–volume loop in Figure 9.10.

53. Identify points *A*, *B*, and *C*.

_____

54. What is the PIP?

_____

55. What is the tidal volume?

_____

56. Why does the loop begin and end at 5 cm $H_2O$?

_____

57. What happens to a pressure–volume loop when lung compliance decreases during VC-CMV?

_____

58. What happens to a pressure–volume loop when lung compliance decreases during PC-CMV?

_____

59. What causes the pressure–volume loop to widen or bulge?

_____

For Questions 60 through 65, refer to the pressure–volume loops in Figure 9.11.

60. What type of breath does loop *A* represent?

_____

61. In which direction does loop *A* move? Why?

_____

62. What type of breath does loop *B* represent?

_____

63. In which direction does loop *B* move? Why?

_____

64. The set flow is 45 L/min; calculate the $R_{aw}$.

_____

65. The difference between the inspiratory and expiratory curves on a volume–pressure loop is called

_____ .

For Questions 66 through 69, refer to the flow–volume loop in Figure 9.12.

66. In which direction does this loop move?

_____

67. What type of flow waveform is represented?

_____

68. The set inspiratory flow rate is _____, and the peak expiratory flow rate is _____.

69. What is the tidal volume?

_____

70. What can cause the expiratory side of a flow–volume loop to end at a volume above zero?

_____

71. What can cause a gap between the inspiratory side and expiratory side on the zero intercept of the *y*-axis (flow) of a flow–volume loop?

_____

## CRITICAL THINKING QUESTIONS

For Questions 1 through 8, refer to the graphs in Figure 9.13.

1. What mode of ventilation is being delivered?

_____

2. Is this patient assisting?

_____

3. What are the total cycle time, $T_I$, expiratory time, and set rate?

_____

_____

4. Describe the problem that is noticeable on the pressure–time curve.

_____

5. Describe the two problems that are noticeable on the volume–time curve.

_____

_____

6. Describe the problem that is noticeable on the flow–time curve.

_____

_____

_____

7. Taking into consideration the three scalars, what is causing these waveform problems?

_____

_____

_____

_____

8. What can be done to eliminate the cause of these problems?

_____

_____

_____

## CASE STUDIES

### Case Study 1

A 68-year-old woman who is 6 feet tall and weighs 120 lbs. was admitted through the emergency department with crushing chest pain. The patient has a history of COPD. Cardiac angiography was performed, and the patient subsequently underwent coronary artery bypass surgery. She now is in the cardiovascular intensive care unit (ICU) receiving mechanical ventilation. Figure 9.14 shows a current pressure–volume loop for this patient.

1. What accounts for the shape of this loop?

_____

_____

_____

2. Is the patient triggering the ventilator? Explain.

_____

_____

_____

3. What is the set tidal volume?

_____

_____

_____

_____

4. What is the PIP?

_____

_____

_____

_____

5. How should the ventilator settings be changed at this time?

_____

_____

_____

_____

_____

_____

## *Case Study 2*

You are the respiratory therapist in the ICU of a large municipal hospital. During rounds, you note the pressure–volume loop in Figure 9.15 for one of your patients.

1. What type of breath is represented?

_____

2. What does the portion of the loop labeled *A* represent?

_____

3. What does the portion of the loop labeled *B* represent?

_____

4. This type of loop moves in which direction?

_____

5. Has PS been set for this patient? Explain.

_____

_____

_____

At the next patient-ventilator system check for this individual, you note the pressure–volume loop shown in Figure 9.16.

6. What type of ventilatory support is the patient receiving?

_____

7. Is the patient making some inspiratory effort?

_____

8. What ventilator adjustment is most appropriate for this patient at this time? Why?

_____

_____

You change the graphic display and now see the graph shown in Figure 9.17.

9. What data can be obtained from this loop?

_____

_____

An hour later, you receive an urgent page to come to this patient. Figure 9.18 shows the current flow–volume loop.

10. Explain the difference between the two flow–volume loops in Figure 9.18.

_____

11. What is the most likely cause of this difference?

_____

12. What therapeutic intervention should you recommend for this patient?

_____

## NBRC-STYLE QUESTIONS

1. In the pressure–time scalar shown in Figure 9.19, line *A* represents which of the following?

    a. Auto-PEEP
    b. $P_{plat}$
    c. PS
    d. Transairway pressure

2. In the pressure–time scalar shown in Figure 9.20, the difference between curve *A* and curve *B* is due to which of the following?

1. Atelectasis
2. Bronchospasm
3. Increased airway secretions
4. Pulmonary edema
    a. 1 and 2
    b. 1 and 3
    c. 2 and 3
    d. 2 and 4

3. Using curve *B* in Figure 9.20, calculate the $R_{aw}$ if the set inspiratory flow rate is 40 L/min.
    a. 0.5 cm $H_2O$/L/s
    b. 2 cm $H_2O$/L/s
    c. 30 cm $H_2O$/L/s
    d. 52 cm $H_2O$/L/s

4. The problem with the pressure–time scalar shown in Figure 9.21 is which of the following?

    a. Patient is actively exhaling
    b. Pressure rise is too rapid
    c. Sensitivity setting is incorrect
    d. Inspiratory pause is too long

5. Correction of the problem identified in Question 4 includes which of the following?
    a. Shorten the $T_I$
    b. Reduce the sensitivity
    c. Adjust the inspiratory slope
    d. Eliminate the inspiratory pause

6. During PSV for a patient with COPD, the respiratory therapist notices a pressure increase toward the end of inspiration on the pressure–time scalar. This phenomenon can be corrected by which of the following?
    a. Shorten the set inspiratory time
    b. Increase the flow cycle percent
    c. Lower the set PS level
    d. Increase the inspiratory flow setting

7. A pressure–volume loop during VC-CMV extends farther to the right and flattens out with which of the following conditions?
   a. Pneumonia
   b. Bronchitis
   c. Asthma
   d. Emphysema
8. A flow–volume loop is incomplete because the volume does not return to zero. This can be caused by which of the following conditions?
   a. Air trapping
   b. Flow starvation
   c. Bronchopleural fistula
   d. Overdistention of alveoli
9. The pressure–time scalar for VC-CMV shown in Figure 9.22 demonstrates which of the following problems?

   a. Flow starvation
   b. Active exhalation
   c. Patient–ventilator dyssynchrony
   d. Incorrect sensitivity setting
10. The flow–volume loop for VC-CMV shown in Figure 9.23 demonstrates which of the following problems?

   a. Atelectasis
   b. Intrinsic PEEP
   c. Flow starvation
   d. Bronchopleural fistula

# 10 Assessment of Respiratory Function

## LEARNING OBJECTIVES

*Upon completion of this chapter, the reader will be able to do the following:*

1. Describe the principle of operation of the pulse oximeter.
2. Identify physiological and technical factors that can influence the accuracy of pulse oximetry readings.
3. Describe how various clinical conditions can affect CO-oximetry, oxygen saturation ($SaO_2$) and pulse oximetry, oxyhemoglobin saturation ($SpO_2$).
4. Discuss the normal components of a capnogram.
5. Give examples of pathophysiological conditions that can alter the contour of the capnogram.
6. Discuss how arterial-to-end-tidal partial pressure of carbon dioxide ($P(a-et)CO_2$) is affected by changes in ventilation-perfusion relationships.
7. Discuss how volumetric $CO_2$ tracings can be used to assess gas exchange during mechanical ventilation.
8. Describe how exhaled nitric oxide measurements can be used in the management of patients with asthma.
9. Explain the theory of operation of transcutaneous $PO_2$ and $PCO_2$ monitors and list the clinical data that should be recorded when making transcutaneous measurements.
10. Provide the respiratory quotient (RQ) value associated with substrate utilization patterns in normal, healthy subjects.
11. Discuss some clinical applications of metabolic monitoring in critically ill patients.
12. Briefly describe devices that are used to measure airway pressures, volumes, and flows during mechanical ventilation.
13. Calculate mean airway pressure, dynamic compliance, static compliance, and airway resistance.
14. Identify pathological conditions that alter lung compliance and airway resistance and measurements of the work of breathing.
15. Define the pressure–time product and discuss its application in the management of mechanically ventilated patients.

**KEY TERMS CROSSWORD PUZZLE**

**Across**

4 The type of pressure measured by occluding the airway during the first 100 ms of a patient's spontaneous inspiration

5 A method of sampling respired gases that extracts gas from the airway through a narrow plastic tube to the measuring chamber, which is located in a separate console

9 The type of dead space free of carbon dioxide

15 Opposition to airflow

17 The type of pressure that reflects alveolar pressure

23 A continuous, noninvasive method of assessing arterial oxygen saturation (two words)

25 Qualitative estimates of exhaled carbon dioxide are made with a _____ detector.

27 Relies on the Beer–Lambert Law

28 The type of hemoglobin that is calculated by dividing the oxyhemoglobin concentration by the concentration of hemoglobin capable of carrying oxygen

29 A breakdown product of heme metabolism that causes a yellow discoloration of the skin

**Down**

1 A term used to describe the movement factor that may affect pulse oximetry readings

2 The difference between gastric and esophageal pressures

3 A complication that can occur with the patient's skin when using transcutaneous monitoring

6 A medical condition that can cause an increase in carbon dioxide production

7 An estimation of energy expenditure from measurements of oxygen consumption and carbon dioxide production is known as _____ calorimetry.

8 A term used to describe states of low perfusion

10 Force times distance

11 Monitoring at the skin surface is known as _____ monitoring.

12 Abnormally low circulating blood volume

13 The type of hemoglobin that has carbon monoxide attached to it

**Down—cont'd**

14 A type of device that samples respired gases whose sampling chamber attaches directly to the endotracheal tube and analysis is performed at the airway

16 The shape of the oxyhemoglobin dissociation curve

18 The measurement of carbon dioxide concentration in respired gases

19 Lung volume achieved for a given amount of applied pressure

20 Instrument accuracy depends on this

21 Absorbs more light at 940 nm

22 Cyclical changes in light transmission allows _____ plethysmography to estimate pulse rate.

24 _____ $CO_2$ monitoring focuses on exhaled $CO_2$ plotted over time, whereas volumetric capnometry focuses on exhaled $CO_2$ plotted relative to exhaled volume (hyphenated word).

26 The type of hemoglobin that absorbs both red and infrared light (abbreviation)

## CHAPTER REVIEW QUESTIONS

1. List five ways to noninvasively monitor the respiratory function of mechanically ventilated patients.
   a. _____
   b. _____
   c. _____
   d. _____
   e. _____

2. List four causes commonly associated with hypoxemic events in mechanically ventilated patients.
   a. _____
   b. _____
   c. _____
   d. _____

3. List four sites where a pulse oximetry sensor can be placed.
   a. _____
   b. _____
   c. _____
   d. _____

4. What are the two principles on which pulse oximetry is based?

5. How is oxyhemoglobin and deoxyhemoglobin differentiated by pulse oximetry?
   _____
   _____
   _____

6. How is pulse rate determined by a pulse oximeter?
   _____
   _____
   _____
   _____
   _____

7. What determines the accuracy of any diagnostic instrument?
   _____

8. Based on the $SpO_2$ reading, when should an arterial blood gas (ABG) be drawn to confirm the patient's oxygen saturation?
   _____

9. Identify four conditions that can influence the accuracy of pulse oximetry readings.
   a. _____
   b. _____
   c. _____
   d. _____

10. List three factors that contribute to low perfusion states in patients.
    a. _____
    b. _____
    c. _____

11. The four types of hemoglobin that adult blood typically contains are:
    a. _____
    b. _____
    c. _____
    d. _____

12. Describe the difference between fractional hemoglobin saturation and functional hemoglobin saturation.
    _____
    _____
    _____
    _____

13. When carboxyhemoglobin (COHb) is present in the blood, what happens to the $SpO_2$?
    _____

14. What medications can cause methemoglobin (MetHb) presence in the blood?
    _____
    _____

15. Describe the effect MetHb has on $SpO_2$ measurements.

_____

_____

16. How can nail polish affect $SpO_2$? What term is used to describe this possible complication?

_____

_____

17. What effect does skin pigmentation have on $SpO_2$?

_____

_____

18. What test is used to determine disparities among $SpO_2$, $SaO_2$, and a patient's clinical presentation?

_____

_____

_____

19. What is the term used to describe the continuous display of carbon dioxide concentrations as a graphic waveform?

_____

20. Describe a specific clinical situation in which chemical capnometer, or colorimetric detector, would be particularly useful.

_____

_____

_____

21. What effect does the presence of water vapor and nitrous oxide have on the accuracy of $CO_2$ measurements?

_____

_____

_____

22. Describe the two methods of gas sampling used by infrared analyzers.
    a. _____

    b. _____

23. What is the normal percentage of $CO_2$ in expired air?

_____

24. Identify and explain the labeled parts of Figure 10.1.

    A. _____

    B. _____

    C. _____

    D. _____

    E. _____

25. What determines the amount of $CO_2$ produced by a patient? Explain.

_____

_____

_____

26. What pathophysiologic conditions can increase or decrease a patient's metabolic rate?

_____

_____

27. For a normal individual, what is the relationship between $PetCO_2$ and $P_aCO_2$?

_____

_____

28. What pathophysiologic conditions cause a decrease in ventilation relative to perfusion, thereby causing a higher than normal $PetCO_2$?

_____

_____

29. Where is the lowest $PetCO_2$ reading in the lungs found?

_____

_____

30. What pathophysiologic conditions cause a decrease in perfusion relative to ventilation, thereby causing a lower than normal $PetCO_2$?

_____

_____

_____

31. List four pathophysiologic conditions that can alter the contour of a capnogram.

    a. _____

    b. _____

    c. _____

    d. _____

32. What do the labeled capnogram waveforms in Figure 10.2 represent?

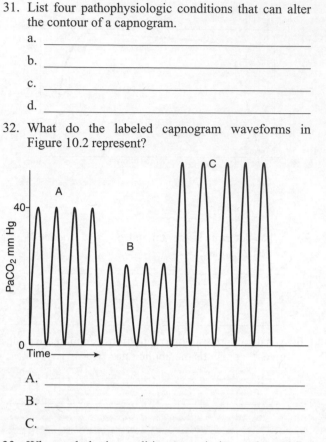

    A. _____

    B. _____

    C. _____

33. What pathologic condition can mimic esophageal intubation identified by capnography?

    _____

    _____

34. Describe a situation that may cause gastric $PCO_2$ to be at almost normal $PetCO_2$ levels.

    _____

    _____

35. What is measuring the $CO_2$ at the end of a forced vital capacity called?

36. What should the $P(a-et)CO_2$ measurement be during normal tidal breathing?

    _____

    _____

37. What do the *x*- and *y*-axis represent in a volumetric $CO_2$ tracing?

    _____

    _____

38. Identify and explain the phases represented by the letters in Figure 10.3, which displays a single breath $CO_2$ curve.

    A. _____

    _____

    B. _____

    _____

    C. _____

39. Label all the blanks in Figure 10.4.

40. Explain the three areas of a volumetric $CO_2$ tracing.

    a. _____

    b. _____

    c. _____

41. What are the four major events that influence the way $CO_2$ is exhaled through the lungs?

    a. _____

    b. _____

    c. _____

    d. _____

42. How can trending $VCO_2$ be used during the weaning process?

    _____

    _____

    _____

    _____

43. Why is the monitoring of exhaled NO useful in the management of severe asthma?

_____

_____

_____

44. What type of electrode is used in a transcutaneous oxygen monitor?

_____

_____

45. Why is the transcutaneous oxygen probe heated?

_____

_____

_____

46. Describe a patient population that is best suited for transcutaneous oxygen monitoring.

_____

_____

47. List five causes of erroneous $PtcO_2$ readings.

a. _____

b. _____

c. _____

d. _____

e. _____

48. What type of electrode is used for transcutaneous carbon dioxide measurements?

_____

49. What effect does heating the transcutaneous carbon dioxide probe have on the measurements?

_____

_____

50. How often should the transcutaneous electrode and sensor membrane be changed?

_____

_____

51. What steps should be taken when placing a transcutaneous electrode on the patient's skin?

_____

_____

_____

_____

52. What are the high and low values for a 2-point calibration of a transcutaneous oxygen monitor?

53. What are the high and low values for a 2-point calibration of a transcutaneous carbon dioxide monitor?

54. List the clinical data that should be documented when making transcutaneous measurements.

_____

_____

_____

_____

55. How often should a transcutaneous sensor be repositioned?

_____

56. What device is most commonly used to perform indirect calorimetry?

_____

57. Describe the major components of an indirect calorimeter.

_____

_____

_____

_____

_____

_____

58. What position should the patient be in and for how long before making an indirect calorimetry measurement?

_____

_____

59. To obtaining indirect calorimetry readings, what should the room temperature range be?

60. Why is a urinary nitrogen level necessary for calculating the energy expenditure?

_____

_____

_____

61. What is the energy expenditure (EE) of a normal healthy adult?

_____

62. When does a hypermetabolic state exists? When does a hypometabolic state exists?

63. List seven conditions that cause hypermetabolic states and five conditions that cause hypometabolic states.

   _____

   _____

   _____

   _____

   _____

   _____

   _____

   _____

   _____

   _____

   _____

   _____

64. What is the RQ range for a healthy adult consuming a typical American diet?

   _____

65. What is the RQ for feedings of large amounts of glucose and for prolonged starvation?

66. When $CO_2$ production increases, what happens to the respiratory quotient?

   _____

67. How can diet influence a patient's failure to wean from mechanical ventilatory support?

   _____

   _____

   _____

   _____

68. What are the devices used to measure airway pressures in the current generation of adult and neonatal ventilators called?

69. Which flow-measuring device can be used to detect bidirectional flow?

   _____

70. What are some potential causes for increases in peak inspiratory pressure (PIP)?

   _____

   _____

71. What is the formula for calculating mean airway pressure?

   _____

72. What is the term used to describe the work to overcome the normal elastic and resistive forces plus the work to overcome a disease process affecting normal workloads in the lung and thorax?

73. List five factors that increase the extrinsic work of breathing.

   a. _____

   b. _____

   c. _____

   d. _____

   e. _____

74. What is the mathematical formula for the work of breathing?

   _____

75. Describe how increases in the airway resistance will affect the results of measurements of the work of breathing.

   _____

   _____

   _____

76. How can a decrease in the static compliance affect the patient's work of breathing?

   _____

   _____

   _____

77. List five pathologic conditions that are associated with decreases in lung compliance.

   a. _____

   b. _____

   c. _____

   d. _____

   e. _____

78. What condition is associated with reductions in both $C_{STAT}$ and $C_{DYN}$?

   _____

   _____

79. What pathologic conditions are associated with increases in airway resistance?

   _____

   _____

   _____

80. What is transdiaphragmatic pressure and how is it measured?

   _____

   _____

   _____

81. What is the pressure–time product?

_____

_____

_____

_____

82. What is occlusion pressure, and how is it measured?

_____

_____

_____

_____

3. What effect does cardiac arrest and decreased cardiac output have on $CO_2$ detection?

_____

_____

_____

_____

_____

_____

## CRITICAL THINKING QUESTIONS

1. Why does pulse oximetry become unreliable when dysfunctional hemoglobins (COHb and MetHb) are present in a patient's blood?

_____

_____

_____

_____

_____

2. When trying to use a finger probe for pulse oximetry, the respiratory therapist finds that pulse rate and the electrocardiogram monitor are not consistent and there is no $SpO_2$ reading. The patient does not have on nail polish. What are the two most likely causes of this problem, and what could be done to correct them?

_____

_____

_____

4. Given the following information, determine whether the patient is in a normal, hypermetabolic, or hypometabolic state. The patient is a 48-year-old female, weight 170 pounds, height 5 feet 7 inches, measured $CO_2$ production is 380 mL/min, and oxygen consumption is 420 mL/min.

_____

_____

_____

_____

_____

_____

_____

_____

_____

## CASE STUDIES

### Case Study 1

A respiratory therapist is assessing a patient receiving mechanical ventilatory support in the intensive care unit. The pulse oximeter attached to the patient is reading an $SpO_2$ of 74%. The patient's $F_IO_2$ is set at 0.40.

1. Is the pulse oximeter reading accurate? Why or why not?

_____

_____

2. The patient's physician asks the respiratory therapist for a recommendation as to which laboratory studies to order to clarify or confirm the pulse oximeter reading. What studies are appropriate for this patient at this time?

_____

_____

## Case Study 2

A patient is brought to the emergency department following an apartment fire. The patient is brought in receiving oxygen from a nonrebreathing mask. Because there are facial burns, the patient is intubated and placed on mechanical ventilatory support with the $F_IO_2$ set at 0.50. The pulse oximeter is reading 99%.

1. Is the pulse oximeter reading accurate? Why or why not?

   _____

   _____

An ABG analysis shows an oxygen saturation of 95% while receiving an $F_IO_2$ of 0.50.

2. Is this saturation accurate? Why or why not?

   _____

   _____

3. In this situation, what lab test should be suggested and why?

   _____

   _____

## Case Study 3

A patient is in the process of being weaned from mechanical ventilatory support and is in the IMV-VC mode and is being monitored with end-tidal $CO_2$. The respiratory therapist has just decreased the ventilator rate to 4 breaths/min; the set $V_T$ is 500 mL. In Figure 10.5, *A* and *B* show the tracings that occurred after this change.

1. Analyze both the $CO_2$ trend and waveform.
_____
_____

2. What are the possible causes for the $CO_2$ trend?
_____
_____

The respiratory therapist observes the patient using accessory muscles during spontaneous breathing. In addition, there is a decreasing spontaneous tidal volume and increasing spontaneous respiratory rate.

3. How do these findings correlate with the $PetCO_2$ findings?
_____
_____
_____

4. How can the problem be alleviated?
_____

## Case Study 4

A respiratory therapist is monitoring the arterial to maximum end-expiratory $PCO_2$ difference for a patient with chronic obstructive pulmonary disease (COPD), who is receiving mechanical ventilatory support. Over the past 24 hours, the $P(a-et)CO_2$ has increased from 5 to 18 mm Hg.

1. Is this increase expected for a patient with COPD? Why or why not?
_____
_____

2. What would a single breath $CO_2$ curve look like for this situation?
_____
_____
_____

## NBRC-STYLE QUESTIONS

1. A pulse oximeter is generally considered accurate for oxygen saturations greater than which of the following?
   a. 65%
   b. 70%
   c. 75%
   d. 80%
2. A respiratory therapist encounters a patient whose pulse oximetry reading is 73%. The most appropriate action is which of the following?
   a. Change the sensor and move it to a different location.
   b. Contact the patient's physician for further instructions.
   c. Confirm the value with arterial blood CO-oximeter analysis.
   d. Accept the value and record it in the patient's medical record.

3. Which of the following most directly affects the response time of a pulse oximeter?
   a. The type of pulse oximeter
   b. The location of the sensor or probe
   c. The percentage of oxygen saturation
   d. The position of the patient in the bed
4. The oxyhemoglobin concentration divided by the concentration of hemoglobin capable of carrying oxygen determines which of the following?
   a. Dysfunctional hemoglobin
   b. Fractional hemoglobin
   c. Functional hemoglobin
   d. Methemoglobin

5. During rounds, a respiratory therapist encounters a patient who is receiving supplemental oxygen and whose $SpO_2$ is constantly displaying 85%. The respiratory therapist notes that the patient is also receiving dapsone. Which of the following is the most appropriate action to take?
   a. Use an ear lobe probe for more accuracy.
   b. Contact the patient's physician for further instructions.
   c. Confirm the value with arterial blood CO-oximeter analysis.
   d. Accept the value and record it in the patient's medical record.

6. The partial pressure of end-tidal carbon dioxide is read at what point on a capnogram?
   a. During phase 1
   b. End of phase 2
   c. During phase 3
   d. End of phase 4

7. The arterial to maximum expiratory $PCO_2$ gradient will be greatest for a patient with which of the following?
   a. COPD
   b. Asthma
   c. Left-sided heart failure
   d. Pulmonary embolism

8. The most reliable method for ruling out esophageal intubation is which of the following?
   a. Presence of $CO_2$ in the patient's exhaled gas
   b. Presence of condensation in the endotracheal tube
   c. Presence of bilateral breath sounds on auscultation
   d. Increased resistance to squeezing the manual resuscitator bag

9. Most likely, cardiac arrest will cause a colorimetric $CO_2$ detector to display which of the following?
   a. Less than 1% $CO_2$
   b. 1% to -2% $CO_2$
   c. 2% to -5% $CO_2$
   d. Greater than 5% $CO_2$

10. A respiratory therapist is called to the bedside of a patient who is being transcutaneously monitored for $PO_2$ and $PCO_2$. The signal is drifting and will not stabilize during calibration. The most appropriate action includes which of the following?
    1. Recalibrate the monitor with 15 and 20% $CO_2$.
    2. Clean the electrode and change the sensor membrane.
    3. Remove the excess electrolyte solution from the electrode surface.
    4. Add a drop of electrolyte solution to the electrode surface.
    a. 1 and 2 only
    b. 1 and 3 only
    c. 2 and 4 only
    d. 3 and 4 only

11. A difficult-to-wean patient with COPD has an RQ of 0.98. The most likely cause of this patient's inability to be weaned is which of the following?
    a. Reliance on lipid metabolism is causing hypoxemia.
    b. Lipogenesis is causing the patient to retain $CO_2$.
    c. A highly restricted carbohydrate metabolism is generating hypoxia.
    d. Excessive carbohydrates are overloading the patient's ventilatory reserve.

12. The tracing of a slow-speed capnograph is not returning to zero every exhalation. The most likely cause of this finding is which of the following?
    a. The $F_IO_2$ was decreased.
    b. The patient is hyperventilating.
    c. $CO_2$ is being rebreathed.
    d. The capnograph needs to be recalibrated.

13. A respiratory therapist monitoring a patient receiving mechanical ventilatory support finds that, over the past 2 hours, the patient's PIP is increasing but the static pressure has remained stable. Which of the following could cause this?
    a. Atelectasis
    b. Pneumothorax
    c. Retained secretions
    d. Right mainstem intubation

14. Which of the following will increase intrinsic work of breathing?
    a. Bronchospasm
    b. Endotracheal tube
    c. Machine sensitivity
    d. Heat moisture exchanger

15. Figure 10.6 is indicative of which of the following?

    a. Mechanical breath with little work of breathing
    b. Spontaneous breath under normal circumstances
    c. Spontaneous breath with high impedance to breathing
    d. Patient breathing through a freestanding continuous positive airway pressure system

# 11 Hemodynamic Monitoring

## LEARNING OBJECTIVES

*Upon completion of this chapter, the reader will be able to do the following:*

1. Discuss how changes in heart rate, preload, contractility, and afterload can alter cardiac function and cardiac output.
2. Identify indicators of left ventricular preload, contractility, and afterload.
3. Name the major components of a hemodynamic monitoring system.
4. Explain the proper technique for insertion and maintenance of a systemic arterial line, and list the most common complications that can occur with this type of monitoring system.
5. Describe the procedures for insertion and placement of a central venous line, and list the potential complications associated with these devices.
6. Interpret the waveforms generated during the insertion of a pulmonary artery catheter.
7. Calculate arterial and venous oxygen content, cardiac output, cardiac index, stroke index, cardiac cycle time, left ventricular stroke work index, right ventricular stroke work index, and pulmonary and systemic vascular resistance.
8. List normal values for measured and derived hemodynamic variables.
9. Describe the most common complications associated with pulmonary artery catheterization and discuss strategies that can be used to minimize these complications.
10. Compare the effects of spontaneous and mechanical ventilation breathing on hemodynamic values.
11. Define the following terms: incisura, pulse pressure, stroke index, stroke work, systemic vascular resistance, pulmonary vascular resistance, ejection fraction.
12. Explain how measurements of pulmonary artery occlusion pressure can be used to evaluate the left ventricular function.
13. Differentiate between cardiogenic and noncardiogenic pulmonary edema using hemodynamic parameters.
14. From a patient case, describe how hemodynamic monitoring can be used in the diagnosis and treatment of selected cases of critically ill patients.

**KEY TERMS CROSSWORD PUZZLE**

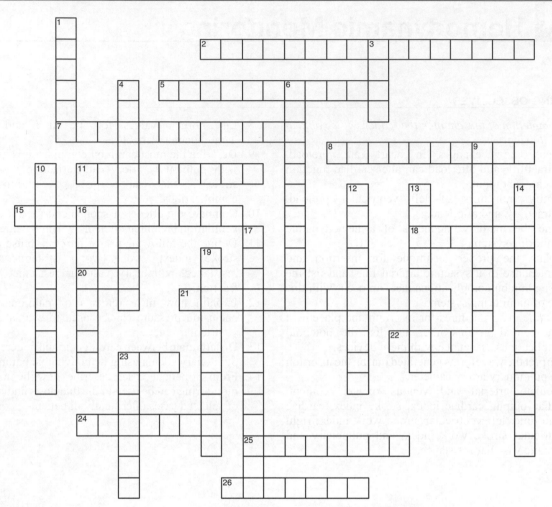

**Across**

2 Ratio of the stroke volume to the ventricular end-diastolic volume (two words)
5 Type of pressure exerted by a fluid while it is at a standstill
7 Type of pressure exerted by a fluid while it is in motion
8 Fluid flowing in the opposite direction
11 One of the atrioventricular valves
15 HRs less than 60 beats/min
18 Valve between the left atrium and left ventricle
20 The afterload that the left ventricle must overcome to eject blood into the systemic circulation (abbreviation)
21 Type of catheter line that is inserted into the right atrium (two words)
22 Another name for pulmonary capillary wedge pressure (abbreviation)
23 The afterload that the right ventricle must overcome to eject blood into the pulmonary circulation (abbreviation)
24 A pulmonary artery catheter floats because of this
25 Small negative deflection on the aortic and pulmonary artery tracing
26 Contraction that causes ejection of blood from the heart

**Down**

1 The unit for pulmonary artery catheter size
3 Principle used to calculate the cardiac output
4 Quantification of the amount of pressure generated by the heart during systole (two words)
6 HRs greater than 100 beats/min
9 Impedance that the left and right ventricles must overcome to eject blood into the great vessels
10 Stroke volume divided by body surface area (two words)
12 Work done by the ventricle to eject a volume of blood into the aorta (two words)
13 Both the aortic and pulmonary valves are this type of valve
14 Difference between the systolic and diastolic pressures (two words)
16 Cardiac relaxation and filling
17 Pumping strength of the heart
19 A type of electrical bridge used in pressure transducers
23 Filling pressure of the ventricle at the end of ventricular diastole

**CHAPTER REVIEW QUESTIONS**

1. List four common invasive hemodynamic measurements.

   a. _____

   b. _____

   c. _____

   d. _____

2. What is the primary indication for hemodynamic monitoring?

   _____

3. When the heart rate is 90 beats/min, what is the length of one cardiac cycle?

   _____

4. What typically causes a retrograde flow in the heart?

   _____

5. Define *afterload*.

   _____

   _____

6. What resistance must the left ventricle overcome to pump blood systemically?

   _____

7. What resistance must the right ventricle overcome to pump blood to the lungs?

   _____

   _____

   _____

8. During atrial systole, which heart valves are open and which are closed?

   _____

   _____

9. What is the term used to describe pressure exerted while a fluid is (a) in motion and (b) not in motion?

   a. _____

   b. _____

10. Where should a transducer be placed to measure accurately?

   _____

11. What happens to the pressure measurement if the transducer is (a) higher than the catheter tip and (b) lower than the catheter tip?

   a. _____

   b. _____

12. What four main factors influence the outputs of the right and left ventricle?

   a. _____

   b. _____

   c. _____

   d. _____

13. Define *preload*.

   _____

14. Describe how ventricular systole occurs.

   _____

   _____

   _____

   _____

   _____

15. What measurements are used to estimate the right ventricular end-diastolic pressure and left ventricular end-diastolic pressure?

   _____

16. What do systemic vascular and pulmonary vascular resistances reflect?

   _____

   _____

17. List the major components of a hemodynamic monitoring system.

   _____

   _____

   _____

18. What is the mid-thoracic line of the patient is called? What is it used to perform on the transducer?

19. Why is positioning of the transducer important for accurate measurements?

   _____

   _____

   _____

20. Explain the proper technique for the insertion and maintenance of a systemic radial arterial line.

    _____

    _____

    _____

    _____

    _____

    _____

21. What are the potential complications that can occur following placement of an arterial catheter line?

    _____

    _____

22. What type of fluid is used to flush an arterial line? How fast should the flow be set?

    _____

    _____

23. What factors increase the risk of infection with an arterial line?

    _____

    _____

24. What potential problem can occur with prolonged or frequent flushing of an arterial line in a neonate or pediatric patient weighing less than 20 kg?

    _____

25. List the uses of a central venous line.

    _____

    _____

26. When a central venous pressure (CVP) measurement is taken at the end of ventricular diastole, what pressure is being estimated?

    _____

    _____

27. List one of the veins typically used for the insertion of a CVP line.

28. CVP measurements are usually taken during which phase of breathing and in what position?

    _____

29. What are two common problems and potential complications from central venous line insertion?

    _____

    _____

30. What is the normal value range for CVP?

31. What are the pediatric and adult pulmonary artery catheter lengths and available sizes? How are they marked off for insertion purposes?

    _____

    _____

32. How are clots avoided in a pulmonary artery catheter?

    _____

    _____

33. Identify the structures, lettered *A* through *G* in Figure 11.1, on a four-channel pulmonary artery catheter.

a. _____

b. _____

c. _____

d. _____

e. _____

f. _____

g. _____

34. List the insertion sites, both percutaneous and surgical cut-down, for the insertion of a pulmonary artery catheter.

_____

_____

35. List eight complications associated with pulmonary artery catheterization. Include the cause of each complication.

a. _____

b. _____

c. _____

d. _____

e. _____

f. _____

g. _____

h. _____

36. What are the two ways to determine catheter position during insertion?

a. _____

b. _____

37. Trace the insertion of a pulmonary artery catheter from an internal jugular vein to a pulmonary vein. When is the balloon inflated? Into which lung zone should the catheter be placed?

_____

_____

_____

38. Why does the pulmonary artery catheter need to be placed in the particular zone described in Question 37?

_____

_____

_____

39. What are the pressure relationships in each lung zone?

| Zone | Pressure Relationship |
|------|----------------------|
| 1 | _____ |
| 2 | _____ |
| 3 | _____ |

40. What is the volume of an adult pulmonary artery catheter balloon? How long should it be inflated for when measuring pulmonary artery occlusion pressure (PAOP)?

41. Identify the position of the catheter represented by the letters *A* through *D* in Figure 11.2.

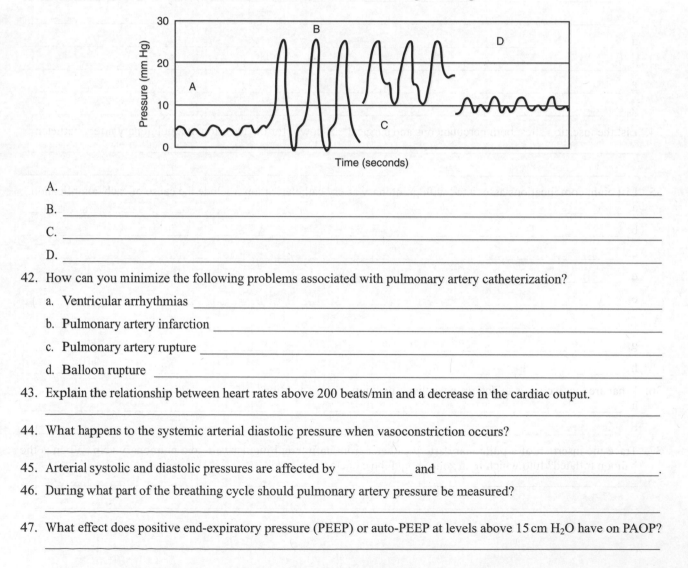

A. _____

B. _____

C. _____

D. _____

42. How can you minimize the following problems associated with pulmonary artery catheterization?

a. Ventricular arrhythmias _____

b. Pulmonary artery infarction _____

c. Pulmonary artery rupture _____

d. Balloon rupture _____

43. Explain the relationship between heart rates above 200 beats/min and a decrease in the cardiac output.

_____

44. What happens to the systemic arterial diastolic pressure when vasoconstriction occurs?

_____

45. Arterial systolic and diastolic pressures are affected by _____ and _____.

46. During what part of the breathing cycle should pulmonary artery pressure be measured?

_____

47. What effect does positive end-expiratory pressure (PEEP) or auto-PEEP at levels above 15 cm $H_2O$ have on PAOP?

_____

48. List three pathologic conditions that increase PVR and subsequently pulmonary artery pressure (PAP).

    a. _____

    b. _____

    c. _____

49. What effect does inhaled nitric oxide have on the pulmonary vasculature?

    _____

    _____

50. Compare the effects of spontaneous breathing to mechanical ventilation as it relates to pulmonary artery pressure.

    _____

    _____

51. Complete the following table with the appropriate hemodynamic values.

| Parameter | Normal Value |
|---|---|
| Arterial blood pressure | _____ |
| Mean arterial pressure | _____ |
| Pulse pressure | _____ |
| CVP | _____ |
| PAP | _____ |
| Pulmonary artery wedge pressure (PAWP) | _____ |

52. Complete the following chart with the formulas used to calculate each value.

| Calculate Value | Formula | Normal Values |
|---|---|---|
| Cardiac output | _____ | _____ |
| Cardiac index | _____ | _____ |
| Stroke index | _____ | _____ |
| Arterial oxygen content | _____ | _____ |
| Mixed venous oxygen content | _____ | _____ |
| SVR | _____ | _____ |
| PVR | _____ | _____ |

53. What are the effects of the following factors on the cardiac output?

| Factor | Effect on Cardiac Output |
|---|---|
| Tachycardia | _____ |
| Beta-adrenergic blockade | _____ |
| Increased parasympathetic tone | _____ |
| Increased preload and contractility | _____ |
| Bradycardia | _____ |
| Decreased parasympathetic tone | _____ |

For Questions 54 through 57, calculate the oxygen content, given the information in each question.

54. $P_aO_2$ 43 mm Hg, $S_aO_2$ 75%, hemoglobin (Hb) 10 g%

    _____

    _____

55. $P_aO_2$ 64 mm Hg, $S_aO_2$ 94%, Hb 13 g%

_____

_____

56. $P_vO_2$ 40 mm Hg, $S_vO_2$ 75%, Hb 15 g%

_____

_____

57. $P_vO_2$ 70 mm Hg, $S_vO_2$ 85%, Hb 16 g%

_____

_____

58. Explain why mixed venous oxygen values decrease when the cardiac output is reduced.

_____

_____

59. What are the two most important factors that influence the vascular resistance? Give examples of each.
    a. _____
    
    b. _____
    
    c. _____

60. What effect does alveolar hypoxia and high intra-alveolar pressures have on PVR?

_____

61. List three mathematically derived indicators of left ventricular contractility.
    a. _____
    
    b. _____
    
    c. _____

## CRITICAL THINKING QUESTIONS

1. Explain how measurements of pulmonary capillary occlusion pressure can be used to evaluate the left ventricular function.

_____

_____

_____

_____

_____

2. Differentiate between cardiogenic and noncardiogenic pulmonary edema using hemodynamic parameters.

_____

_____

_____

_____

_____

_____

_____

3. Define pulse pressure. What conditions can lead to (a) an increased pulse pressure and (b) a decreased pulse pressure?

a. _____

_____

b. _____

_____

_____

## CASE STUDIES

### Case Study 1

A 53-year-old, 6-foot tall, 195-lb man was admitted for head trauma due to a motor vehicle crash. In the operating room, the patient had a craniotomy to relieve pressure. He is currently in the surgical intensive care unit receiving mechanical ventilation with VC-IMV, rate 8, $V_T$ 650 mL, and $F_IO_2$ 0.6. The patient is receiving dobutamine. A pulmonary artery catheter is inserted, and the following information is collected:

| | | |
|---|---|---|
| PAP: 38/20 mm Hg | CVP: 12 mm Hg | HR: 92 beats/min |
| PAWP: 10 mm Hg | BP: 145/68 mm | Hg Hb: 12.6 g% |
| CO: 5.1 L/min | | |

| | Arterial Blood Gas | Mixed Venous Gas |
|---|---|---|
| pH | 7.46 | 7.38 |
| $PCO_2$ | 32 mm Hg | 43 mm Hg |
| $P_aO_2$ | 100 mm Hg | 40 mm Hg |
| $S_aO_2$ | 99% | 75% |

Calculate the following, and indicate whether normal, high, or low:

1. Pulse pressure _____

2. Stroke volume _____

3. Stroke index _____

4. Cardiac index _____

5. Mean arterial pressure _____

6. Mean pulmonary artery pressure _____

7. SVR _____

8. PVR _____

9. $C_aO_2$ _____

10. $C_vO_2$ _____

11. $C(a-v)O_2$ _____

12. $DO_2$ _____

13. $VO_2$ _____

14. RVSW _____

15. RVSWI _____

16. LVSW _____

17. LVSWI _____

18. Comment on the patient data. _____

## Case Study 2

The respiratory therapist is monitoring a patient who is receiving mechanical ventilatory support in one of the intensive care units. Hemodynamic monitoring of this patient is being considered because of patient instability.

1. What aspect of hemodynamic monitoring should the respiratory therapist suggest for this patient?

   _____

   _____

A hemodynamic monitoring system is now in place. The catheter was inserted through the subclavian 1 hour ago. The patient is now exhibiting signs of respiratory distress. Breath sounds are absent on the patient's right side.

2. What complication is most likely causing this clinical situation?

   _____

3. What is the most likely cause of this complication?

   _____

Following correction of the problem, the PAOP was 12 mm Hg. As the day progressed, however, the pressure rose to 15 mm Hg, and then over the next few hours to 19 mm Hg. The pressure has now stabilized at 25 mm Hg.

4. What is the significance of this finding?

   _____

## NBRC-STYLE QUESTIONS

1. The respiratory therapist is assisting a physician inserting a pulmonary artery catheter in a patient when it is noted that a dampened or continuous low-pressure waveform is displayed on the oscilloscope. This indicates which of the following?
   a. The catheter is not wedged.
   b. The balloon is deflated, and the catheter is not wedged.
   c. The balloon may still be inflated, or the catheter may be wedged.
   d. The balloon is deflated, and the catheter has perforated the right ventricle.

2. The PAOP value most indicative of cardiogenic pulmonary edema is which of the following?
   a. 8 mm Hg
   b. 12 mm Hg
   c. 18 mm Hg
   d. 25 mm Hg

3. The pressure measured from the proximal lumen of a pulmonary artery catheter is referred to as:
   a. PAP
   b. RAP
   c. RVP
   d. PAWP

4. Which of the following procedures verifies the position of a pulmonary catheter?
   a. Checking the pressure waveform
   b. Checking the number of centimeters inserted
   c. Obtaining a blood sample through the catheter tip
   d. Obtaining a chest radiograph for catheter tip placement

5. The third lumen of a pulmonary artery catheter is used to measure which of the following?
   a. CO
   b. CVP
   c. PAP
   d. PAOP

6. A low CVP value is indicative of which of the following?
   a. Shock, dehydration, or hemorrhage
   b. Shock, overhydration, or hemorrhage
   c. Hypertension, dehydration, or hypervolemia
   d. Hypertension, overhydration, and hypovolemia

7. Which of the following complications is most common following long-term placement of systemic arterial catheterization?
   a. Hemorrhage and spasm of the artery
   b. Cardiac valve stenosis and prolapse
   c. Arterial laceration and subsequent hemorrhage
   d. Infection and tissue ischemia distal to the catheter

8. The proper location for the distal tip of a central venous catheter is in which of the following?
   a. Left ventricle or aorta
   b. Vena cava or right atrium
   c. Right ventricle or pulmonary artery
   d. Pulmonary artery or pulmonary capillary

9. Which of the following measurements may best estimate the left ventricular preload?
   a. RAP
   b. CVP
   c. PAP
   d. PAOP

10. Which of the following will increase the cardiac index?
    a. Shock
    b. Exercise
    c. Hypovolemia
    d. Cardiac failure

# 12 Methods to Improve Ventilation in Patient–Ventilator Management

## LEARNING OBJECTIVES

*Upon completion of this chapter, the reader will be able to do the following:*

1. Recommend ventilator adjustments to reduce work of breathing and improve ventilation based on patient diagnosis, arterial blood gas results, and ventilator parameters.
2. Calculate the appropriate suction catheter size, length, and amount of suction pressure needed for a specific size endotracheal tube and a patient.
3. Compare the benefits of closed-suction catheters with the open-suction technique.
4. List the pros and cons of instilling normal saline to loosen secretions before suctioning.
5. List the clinical findings used to establish the presence of a respiratory infection.
6. Compare and contrast the protocols for using metered-dose inhalers and small-volume nebulizers during mechanical ventilation.
7. Describe complications associated with using small-volume nebulizers powered by external flowmeters during mechanical ventilation.
8. Discuss the importance of patient-centered mechanical ventilation in the treatment of critically ill patients.
9. Discuss the complications associated with the in-house transport of a mechanically ventilated patient.

**KEY TERMS CROSSWORD PUZZLE**

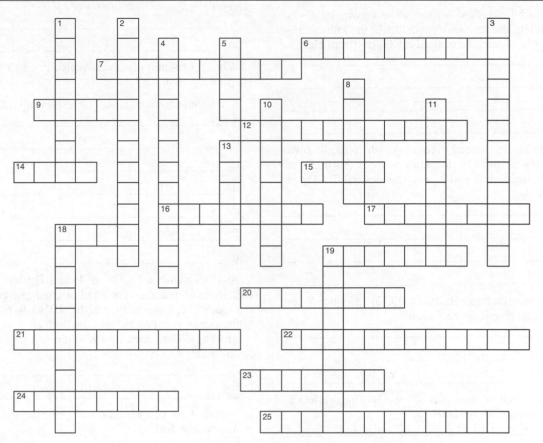

## Across

6 _____ overdose can cause metabolic acidosis.
7 Caused by a medical procedure or treatment
9 Fever, multiple trauma, sepsis, and _____ can increase metabolism and $CO_2$ production.
12 Normal ventilation
14 Medication given to keep pH greater than 7.25 (abbreviation)
15 Type of suctioning that can decrease ventilator-associated pneumonias (VAPs) in intubated patients (abbreviation)
16 $CO_2$ causes vasodilation here
17 Deficient blood flow to the cells
18 Type of aerosol device that delivers puffs of medication (abbreviation)
19 A bag for collecting a patient's exhaled air
20 Rigid tonsil suction tip
21 In pressure-controlled ventilation (PCV), increasing this time will increase the volume delivered without increasing the pressure
22 "Out of step" with the ventilator
23 A fluid filled with cellular debris and protein that accumulates as a result of inflammation
24 Respiratory acidosis indicates that this type of ventilation is not adequate
25 Part of the standard therapy to reduce intracranial pressure

## Down

1 Reduced urinary output
2 Defined as across the pyloric region of the stomach, this type of enteral feeding route reduces the risks of vomiting and aspiration
3 Overhydration causes this effect, which can lead to reduced hemoglobin, hematocrit, and cell counts
4 Procedure for visualizing the bronchi
5 A type of acidosis caused by diabetes, alcoholism, or starvation
8 Suctioning can cause ulceration of the_____.
10 Excessive urinary output
11 Loss of bicarbonate can be caused by _____.
13 A thyroid that is overactive is _____.
18 Hypercapnia used to help prevent lung injury
19 Ventilation without perfusion (two words)

## CHAPTER REVIEW QUESTIONS

1. Calculate the desired $V_T$ when the known $P_aCO_2$ is 55 mm Hg, the known $V_T$ is 500 mL, the known frequency is 14, and the desired $P_aCO_2$ is 40 mm Hg.

_____

_____

_____

2. Calculate the desired frequency when the known $P_aCO_2$ is 65 mm Hg, the known $V_T$ is 600 mL, the known frequency is 12, and the desired $P_aCO_2$ is 50 mm Hg.

_____

_____

_____

3. What three factors can affect $P_aCO_2$ in patients receiving mechanical ventilation?
   a. _____
   b. _____
   c. _____

4. List the three components of an ABG that reflect a patient's ventilatory status.
   a. _____
   b. _____
   c. _____

5. What happens to the $PaCO_2$ and the pH when alveolar ventilation decreases?

_____

_____

6. List six pathologic processes that are associated with acute respiratory acidosis.
   a. _____
   b. _____
   c. _____
   d. _____
   e. _____
   f. _____

7. Explain how volume and pressure affect $P_aCO_2$ and pH?

_____

_____

_____

8. What is the recommended target $V_T$? _____

9. When increasing $V_T$, it is important to maintain $P_{plat}$ of less than what value? _____

10. List two methods of increasing $V_T$ in pressure-control ventilation.
    a. _____
    b. _____

11. What $P_aCO_2$ and pH levels typically characterize respiratory alkalosis?

12. List seven common causes of respiratory alkalosis.
    a. _____
    b. _____
    c. _____
    d. _____
    e. _____
    f. _____
    g. _____

13. A patient with a $P_aCO_2$ of 25 mm Hg and a pH of 7.55 is sedated and ventilated in a volume-controlled mode. The ideal body weight (IBW) is 60 kg. The frequency is set at 18, and the delivered $V_T$ is set at 8 mL/kg. What frequency would result in a $P_aCO_2$ of 40 mm Hg?

_____

_____

14. Explain how you would correct respiratory alkalosis in a patient during:
    a. Volume-controlled ventilation: _____
    b. Pressure-controlled ventilation: _____

15. A patient on VC-CMV has the frequency set at 10, with the total respiratory rate of 20 breaths/min. The $P_aCO_2$ is 25 mm Hg with a pH of 7.52. Will decreasing the set rate correct the respiratory alkalosis? Explain your answer.

_____

_____

16. Referring to Question 15, what modes of ventilation may be more appropriate for this patient? Why?

_____

_____

17. List six common causes of hyperventilation in patients receiving mechanical ventilation.
    a. _____
    b. _____
    c. _____
    d. _____
    e. _____
    f. _____

18. What is the body's physiologic response to a metabolic acidosis?

    _____

    _____

19. List six causes of metabolic acidosis. Give an example of each.

    a. _____

    b. _____

    c. _____

    d. _____

    e. _____

    f. _____

20. What are the pH and bicarbonate levels that typically characterize metabolic acidosis?

    _____

21. List five common causes of metabolic alkalosis.

    a. _____

    b. _____

    c. _____

    d. _____

    e. _____

22. What two formulas are used to predict the change in pressure necessary to achieve a desired $P_aCO_2$?

    a. _____

    b. _____

23. How can mechanical ventilation cause an increase in a patient's dead space?

    _____

    _____

    _____

24. List two examples of pathologic processes that would result in an increase in the physiologic dead space.

    a. _____

    b. _____

25. What is the normal range for the $V_D/V_T$ ratio?

    _____

    _____

26. Calculate the $V_D/V_T$ ratio based on the following information: $V_T = 800\,mL$, $P_aCO_2 = 45\,mm\,Hg$, $P_ECO_2 = 36\,mm\,Hg$.

    _____

    _____

27. List eight clinical disorders that may result in a hypermetabolic state.

    a. _____

    b. _____

    c. _____

    d. _____

    e. _____

    f. _____

    g. _____

    h. _____

28. What effect does hyperventilation have on cerebral blood flow?

    _____

29. Describe permissive hypercapnia.

    _____

    _____

30. What is the effect of permissive hypercapnia on patients with head trauma?

    _____

    _____

31. List the suction pressure ranges for adults, children, and infants.

    _____

    _____

32. What is the maximum length of suction time for an adult?

33. What is the estimated suction catheter size for a 7.0 ET?

    _____

    _____

34. List five indications for the endotracheal suctioning of mechanically ventilated patients with artificial airways according to the American Association or Respiratory Care Clinical Practice Guidelines.

    a. _____

    b. _____

    c. _____

    d. _____

    e. _____

35. Are there any contraindications to suctioning?

    _____

36. List nine indications for the use of closed in-line suctioning.

a. _____

b. _____

c. _____

d. _____

e. _____

f. _____

g. _____

h. _____

i. _____

37. Match the complication with its most likely cause.

**Complication**

_____ Hypoxemia/hypoxia

_____ Tracheal/mucosal trauma

_____ Cardiac/respiratory arrest

_____ Cardiac arrhythmias

_____ Atelectasis

_____ Bronchospasm

_____ Infection

_____ Bleeding

**Cause**

a. Suction pressures

b. Reduction in lung volume

c. Airway trauma

d. Patient or caregiver

e. Hypoxemia/vagal stimulation

f. Extreme response to suctioning and vent disconnect

g. Ventilator disconnect and loss of PEEP

h. Reaction to tracheal stimulation

38. Describe presuctioning and postsuctioning procedures as it relates to $F_IO_2$?

_____

39. List four advantages of closed in-line suction catheter use.

a. _____

b. _____

c. _____

d. _____

40. List five disadvantages of in-line suction catheter use.

a. _____

b. _____

c. _____

d. _____

e. _____

41. List four reasons why silent aspiration and VAP can occur with cuffed ET tubes.

a. _____

b. _____

c. _____

d. _____

42. Describe how silent aspiration and VAP may occur.

_____

_____

_____

43. What is the benefit of using a Hi-Lo Evac ET tube?

_____

_____

_____

44. What pressure should be used with a CASS ET tube?

_____

45. Should you instill saline down the ET before performing endotracheal suctioning? Why or why not?

_____

_____

_____

46. How can ET suctioning be assessed in a patient receiving mechanical ventilation?

_____

_____

_____

47. What parameters should be monitored prior to, during, and after suctioning?

_____

_____

48. Following suctioning of an intubated patient, the respiratory therapist notices that the sputum is rust colored. What is the patient's potential problem?

_____

49. List four patient-related factors that influence aerosol deposition in a mechanically ventilated patient.

a. _____

b. _____

c. _____

d. _____

50. List the four types of aerosol-generating devices that can be used to administer aerosolized medications during mechanical ventilation?

    a. _____

    b. _____

    c. _____

    d. _____

51. Which mode of mechanical ventilation is thought to be more effective for aerosol delivery?

    _____

52. Explain how ventilator tidal volume and respiratory rate affect aerosol delivery.

    _____

    _____

53. What technical problems with the ventilator are associated with the continuous nebulization using an external gas source?

    _____

    _____

    _____

54. Where in the ventilator circuit should the nebulizers be placed?

    _____

    _____

55. What three factors would optimize the aerosol deposition of bronchodilators during noninvasive positive-pressure ventilation?

    a. _____

    b. _____

    c. _____

56. List four positive patient responses to bronchodilator therapy during mechanical ventilation.

    a. _____

    b. _____

    c. _____

    d. _____

57. A mechanically ventilated patient is given albuterol via pMDI. The pretreatment and post-treatment findings are

    Pretreatment: peak inspiratory pressure (PIP) = 32 cm $H_2O$, $P_{plat}$ = 8 cm $H_2O$

    Post-treatment: PIP = 23 cm $H_2O$, $P_{plat}$ = 10 cm $H_2O$

    Was this treatment effective? Why or why not?

    _____

58. What is the goal when performing chest physiotherapy?

    _____

    _____

59. Chest physiotherapy includes which two procedures?

    _____

60. List the sequence of four recommended positions that aid in secretion clearance for ventilated patients.

    a. _____

    b. _____

    c. _____

    d. _____

61. List the possible hazards of performing chest physiotherapy on patients requiring mechanical ventilation:

    _____

    _____

    _____

62. List the three channels found in a flexible fiberoptic bronchoscope and the purpose for each.

    a. _____

    b. _____

    c. _____

63. What medication can be given to a ventilated patient prior to a bronchoscopy to reduce secretion production and block the vagal response?

    _____

64. What type of patient problem should be suspected when the patient's cardiac output and renal output are decreased and the pulmonary artery occlusions pressure is increased?

    _____

65. What is considered normal urinary output?

    _____

66. What effect can positive-pressure ventilation have on urinary output?

    _____

67. What effect does fluid balance have on blood cell counts?

    _____

    _____

68. Describe the objective of patient-centered mechanical ventilation.

    _____

    _____

69. Which ventilator parameters can be adjusted by the respiratory therapist to improve patient comfort?

_____

_____

_____

_____

70. What equipment is needed for the in-house transport of a mechanically ventilated patient?

_____

_____

71. What capabilities should a transport ventilator have to ensure patient safety?

_____

_____

72. List four contraindications to the in-house transport of a mechanically ventilated patient.

a. _____

b. _____

c. _____

d. _____

## CRITICAL THINKING QUESTIONS

1. A patient is being ventilated in a volume-controlled mode. The set $V_T$ is 700 mL with a frequency of 10. The $P_{plat}$ equals 45 cm $H_2O$, and the $P_aCO_2$ equals 60 mm Hg. The physician would like to reduce the $P_aCO_2$ to 40 mm Hg, but does not want to increase the $V_T$ because of the high $P_{plat}$. What can the therapist do to decrease the level of $P_aCO_2$ to 40 mm Hg?

_____

_____

_____

_____

2. A postsurgical patient who suffered trauma following multiple surgical procedures is septic with a fever of 104° F. The patient is being maintained in a volume-controlled mode of ventilation. The $V_T$ is 800 mL, with a set frequency of 15, and the patient is triggering to 25 breaths/min. An ABG reveals a $P_aCO_2$ of 38 mm Hg and a $P_aO_2$ of 42 mm Hg. Why does the patient have a normal $P_aCO_2$ with a minute ventilation of 20 L/min?

_____

_____

_____

_____

3. A patient in respiratory distress was intubated and placed on pressure-control ventilation with a PEEP level of +5 cm $H_2O$. Soon after, the patient's cardiac output decreases from 6 to 4.5 L/min. What can the therapist do to help determine what was responsible for the decrease in the cardiac output?

_____

_____

_____

_____

## CASE STUDIES

### Case Study 1

A patient is being ventilated with VC-CMV, rate is 12 breaths/min, $V_T$ is 700 mL, $F_IO_2$ is 0.5, and PEEP is 5 cm $H_2O$. The total rate is 25 breaths/min. The pH is 7.52, $P_aCO_2$ is 30 mm Hg, and $P_aO_2$ is 45 mm Hg. When the set frequency was reduced to 10 in an attempt to correct the respiratory alkalosis, the total rate remained at 25. An attempt at decreasing the $V_T$ resulted in an increase in the total rate.

1. What can the therapist do to address the respiratory alkalosis for this patient?

_____

_____

_____

### Case Study 2

A 100-kg (IBW) patient is receiving PCV with a set pressure of 20 cm $H_2O$ at a frequency of 12 breaths/min. The flow rate reaches zero before the beginning of exhalation. The exhaled volume is 550 mL, $P_aCO_2$ is 65 mm Hg, and pH is 7.29. The physician requests that the patient's $P_aCO_2$ be decreased to 45 mm Hg.

1. What would be the most effective means of reducing the patient's $P_aCO_2$?
   _____

2. What parameter change would result in the desired $P_aCO_2$ of 45 mm Hg?
   _____
   _____
   _____
   _____
   _____

### Case Study 3

A patient with poor compliance is being ventilated in a pressure-controlled mode. The PEEP level is set at 10 cm $H_2O$ with an $F_IO_2$ of 60. The patient is manually ventilated with 100% $O_2$ before suctioning. When the ventilator is disconnected from the ET tube and the therapist begins the procedure, there is a rapid drop in $O_2$ saturation and a marked increase in the heart rate.

1. What is the possible cause of the problem?
   _____
   _____
   _____

2. What can the therapist do to alleviate the situation?
   _____
   _____

### NBRC-STYLE QUESTIONS

1. Which of the following aerosol delivery devices will affect ventilator function when used?
   a. pMDI
   b. USN
   c. SVN
   d. VMN
2. Permissive hypercapnia may be beneficial for a patient with which of the following?
   a. High $P_{plat}$
   b. Intracranial lesion
   c. Pulmonary hypertension
   d. Head trauma
3. A patient requiring mechanical ventilation has an 8-mm ET in place. The patient requires frequent suctioning and a 10-French catheter is being used. The respiratory therapist should recommend which of the following?
   a. Instill saline with every suctioning procedure
   b. A suction frequency of every 2 hours
   c. Increase the suction pressure to $-180$ mm Hg
   d. Changing to a size 12-French catheter
4. Which of the following statements pertaining to the Hi-Lo Evac ET is true?
   a. The tube has a suction port at the level of the ET cuff.
   b. The continuous suction pressure should be set at $-30$ cm $H_2O$.
   c. The device can reduce the incidence of nosocomial pneumonias.
   d. All patients should have this type of ET tube in place.
5. An 85-kg male (IBW) patient is being ventilated with VC-CMV, $f = 12$ breaths/min, ans $V_T = 450$ mL. The patient's ABG results reveal $PaCO_2 = 55$ mm Hg. Which of the following changes should be made to the ventilator to reduce the patient's $PaCO_2$ to 40 mm Hg?
   a. Increase the $V_T$ to 620 mL.
   b. Decrease the $V_T$ to 400 mL.
   c. Increase the rate to 18 breaths/min.
   d. Decrease the rate to 10 breaths/min.

6. A patient with a white blood cell count of $13.3 \times 10_3$/ mcL is coughing up moderate amounts of yellow secretions. Physical examination reveals decreased breath sounds and dullness to percussion. These findings are consistent with which of the following?
   a. Airway trauma
   b. Pulmonary embolism
   c. Pneumonia
   d. Pulmonary edema

7. Which of the following can cause an increase in the physiologic dead space?
   1. Pulmonary embolism
   2. An increase in VT
   3. Low cardiac output
   4. High alveolar pressures
   a. 1 only
   b. 1 and 2
   c. 1, 3, and 4
   d. 1, 2, 3, and 4

8. A patient receiving mechanical ventilation should not be transported under which of the following conditions?
   1. Patient is hemodynamically unstable.
   2. It is not possible to monitor cardiac function.
   3. Patient is nasally intubated.
   4. Patient has multiple IV lines.
   a. 1 only
   b. 1 and 2
   c. 1, 3, and 4
   d. 1, 2, 3, and 4

9. Methods for managing the ventilatory status of a patient with unilateral lung disease include which of the following?
   1. Use of a double-lumen ET
   2. Instillation of normal saline before suctioning
   3. Bronchodilator therapy via a small volume nebulizer
   4. Position the patient laterally so that the good lung is dependent
   a. 1 only
   b. 1, 2, and 3
   c. 1, 2, 3, and 4
   d. 1 and 4

10. The concept of *patient-centered mechanical ventilation* includes which of the following?
    a. Determining the patient comfort level
    b. Maintaining a $P_aO_2$ greater than 60 mm Hg
    c. Maintaining the $P_{plat}$ less than 40 cm $H_2O$
    d. Determining the nutritional needs

# 13 Improving Oxygenation and Management of Acute Respiratory Distress Syndrome

*Upon completion of this chapter, the reader will be able to do the following:*

1. Calculate a desired $F_IO_2$ required to achieve a desired $P_aO_2$, based on current ventilator settings and blood gases.
2. Calculate a patient's pulmonary shunt fraction.
3. Identify indications and contraindications for continuous positive airway pressure (CPAP) and positive end-expiratory pressure (PEEP).
4. List the primary goal of PEEP and the conditions in which high levels of PEEP are most often used.
5. Describe the most appropriate method for establishing an optimum level of PEEP for a patient with acute respiratory distress syndrome (ARDS) using a recruitment–derecruitment maneuver and the deflection point (lower inflection point during deflation or derecruitment).
6. Explain the effects of PEEP/CPAP therapy on a patient with a unilateral lung disease. Describe the problems associated with initiating PEEP in a patient with an untreated pneumothorax.
7. Recommend adjustments in PEEP and ventilator settings based on the physical assessment of the patient, arterial blood gases (ABGs), and ventilator parameters.
8. Compare static compliance, hemodynamic data, and ABGs as indicators of an optimal PEEP.
9. Identify from patient assessment and ABGs when it is appropriate to change from CPAP to mechanical ventilation with PEEP.
10. Identify the severity of ARDS using the $P_aO_2/F_IO_2$ ratio.
11. Recommend an appropriate tidal volume (VT) setting for a patient with ARDS.
12. Identify the maximum plateau pressure ($P_{plat}$) value to use for patients with ARDS.
13. Identify the criteria that should be used to liberate a patient from PEEP or CPAP.
14. Recommend a PEEP setting based on the inflection point on the deflation curve using the pressure–volume loop for a patient with ARDS.
15. Describe the procedure for prone positioning in ventilated patients with ARDS.
16. List potential problems associated with placing the patient in a prone position during mechanical ventilation.
17. Discuss several theories that describe how prone positioning improves ventilation-perfusion in ARDS.

# KEY TERMS CROSSWORD PUZZLE

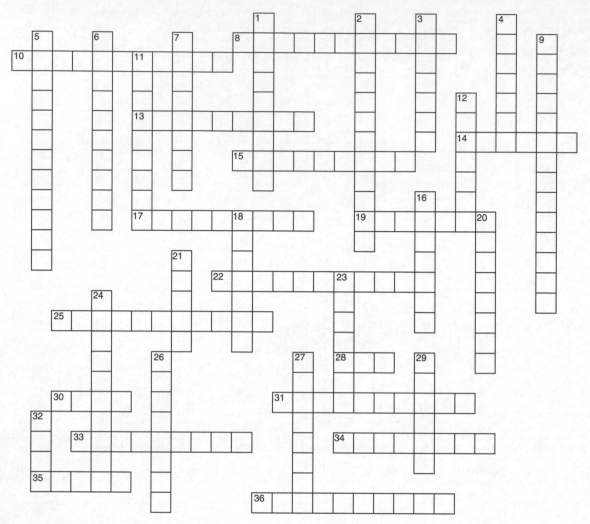

## Across

8 Hemorrhaging or dehydration can cause this
10 A maneuver used to open collapsed alveoli
13 The phase of ARDS characterized by inflammation and alveolar filling
14 Lung units
15 Point that occurs when a large number of lung units collapse quickly
17 Zone 3 of the lungs is _____.
19 The PEEP level that has the maximum benefit
22 Type of pulmonary edema due to congestive heart failure (CHF)
25 Partial or complete collapse of the previously expanded areas of a lung producing a shrunken, airless state
28 The point on a static pressure–volume curve where the slope of the line changes significantly (abbreviation)
30 _____-billed appearance of pressure–volume curve shows over distention
31 Injury to the lung parenchyma caused by excessive pressures in the lungs
33 _____ alveolitis is the second phase of ARDS
34 Toward the head area
35 Perfusion without ventilation
36 A type of hypoxia caused by cyanide poisoning

## Down

1 A type of inflammatory mediator
2 Creates a resistance to gas flow through an orifice (two words)
3 Alter $F_IO_2$ depending on oxygen saturation
4 Pressure that pulls fluid out of tissues
5 High thoracic pressures can reduce this (two words)
6 Material produced by type II pneumocytes
7 Has blood flowing through its capillaries
9 Keep $F_IO_2$ low to avoid this (two words)
11 A resistor that maintains pressure independent of flow
12 A pressure measurement taken during positive-pressure ventilation (PPV) after a breath has been delivered to the patient and before exhalation has begun
16 Material from which some CPAP masks are made
18 Type of PV loop obtained during gas flow
20 Chemical that causes inflammation
21 A Drager ventilator
23 A Hamilton ventilator
24 Point that occurs where a large number of lung units collapse quickly
26 Cellular death
27 Breath sound indicative of pulmonary edema
29 Toward the base of the spine
32 A specific clinical disorder that benefits from PEEP (abbreviation)

## CHAPTER REVIEW QUESTIONS

1. Explain the difference between hypoxemia and hypoxia.

2. What information does the measurement of oxygen delivery provide?

3. What are the formulas used for calculating oxygen delivery and consumption?

4. How often should the $F_IO_2$ be monitored on adult and pediatric patients receiving mechanical ventilation?

5. How soon after a change in the $F_IO_2$ is made can an ABG be drawn?

6. At what level should the $F_IO_2$ be maintained to help prevent the complications of oxygen toxicity?

7. By what mechanism can breathing 100% oxygen contribute to hypoxemia?

8. What is the target range for $P_aO_2$ when administering supplemental oxygen for most adult patients?

9. Your patient is receiving an $F_IO_2$ of 0.8, yet their $P_aO_2$ remains low. What could be happening?

10. What formula is used to calculate the desired $F_IO_2$ necessary to obtain a desired $P_aO_2$?

11. Thirty minutes after initiating pressure-targeted ventilation, an ABG is drawn with the following results: pH = 7.43, $P_aCO_2$ = 43 mm Hg, $P_aO_2$ = 50 mm Hg. The $F_IO_2$ is set at 75%, with a PEEP level of 5 cm $H_2O$. What $F_IO_2$ is needed to achieve a desired $P_aO_2$ of 60 mm Hg?

12. What is the significance of calculating a patient's pulmonary shunt?

13. What is the classic shunt equation for calculating the patient's pulmonary shunt?

14. Given the following information, calculate the patient's pulmonary shunt fraction: $Cc'O_2$ = 20.4 vol%, $CaO_2$ = 19.8 vol%, $C'O_2$ = 13.4 vol%

15. Define mean airway pressure (*Paw*).

16. List five factors that affect *Paw* during PPV.
    a.
    b.
    c.
    d.
    e.

17. How does increasing *Paw* increase $P_aO_2$ in the presence of ventilation/perfusion abnormalities and/or diffusion defects?

18. List four methods of increasing *Paw*:
    a.
    b.
    c.
    d.

19. What are four goals of PEEP/CPAP therapy?
    a. _____
    b. _____
    c. _____
    d. _____

20. Explain the difference between the terms PEEP and CPAP.
    _____
    _____
    _____

21. How is PEEP applied to the lungs during mechanical ventilation and what is the desired physiologic result?
    _____
    _____
    _____

22. List four devices capable of applying PEEP/CPAP to the airway
    a. _____
    b. _____
    c. _____
    d. _____

23. List the patient criteria necessary for placing a patient on mask CPAP.
    _____
    _____
    _____

24. List four hazards associated with the use of mask CPAP.
    a. _____
    b. _____
    c. _____
    d. _____

25. List six indications for PEEP therapy.
    a. _____
    b. _____
    c. _____
    d. _____
    e. _____
    f. _____

26. What is the difference between physiologic PEEP and therapeutic PEEP?
    _____
    _____
    _____
    _____

27. What is optimal PEEP?
    _____
    _____
    _____
    _____

28. What physiologic parameters are monitored while determining optimal PEEP?
    _____
    _____
    _____
    _____

29. During volume-controlled ventilation, the PEEP level is set at +5 cm $H_2O$ and the $P_{peak}$ is 42 cm $H_2O$. After the PEEP is increased to 10 cm $H_2O$, the $P_{peak}$ is now measured at 48 cm $H_2O$. Has the patient's condition worsened? What caused the increase in $P_{peak}$?
    _____
    _____
    _____

30. What happens within the independent zones of the lungs with ARDS when the PEEP is applied in increasing levels? How can this be avoided?
    _____
    _____
    _____

31. How does positive pressure benefit patients with acute pulmonary edema due to CHF?
    _____
    _____
    _____

32. When PEEP is indicated, how soon should it be initiated? Explain your answer.
    _____
    _____
    _____

33. List three specific clinical disorders that may benefit from the use of PEEP/CPAP.

    a. _____

    b. _____

    c. _____

34. What effects will PEEP have on a patient with an untreated pneumothorax?

    _____

    _____

    _____

35. Why is PEEP therapy not always beneficial to patients with emphysema?

    _____

    _____

36. List five criteria that may indicate that a patient is ready for a trial reduction of PEEP.

    a. _____

    b. _____

    c. _____

    d. _____

    e. _____

37. In your own words, define ARDS.

    _____

    _____

    _____

38. What onset of time does the *Berlin Definition* of ARDS specify?

    _____

39. Identify the two phases of ARDS and the characteristics of each.

    a. _____

    b. _____

40. Why does pulmonary edema develop in the ARDS patient?

    _____

41. How should fluid be managed in the ARDS patient?

    _____

42. What are the two categories of ARDS?

    a. _____

    b. _____

43. Define the following terms related to the computed tomography in an ARDS patient.

    a. Ground glass opacification: _____

    b. Consolidation: _____

    c. Reticular pattern: _____

44. What are the basic points that should be kept in mind when managing ventilated patients with ARDS using an open-lung or lung-protective strategy?

    a. _____

    b. _____

    c. _____

    d. _____

    e. _____

    f. _____

    g. _____

45. Explain how a normal lung can become damaged during the management of ARDS.

    _____

46. What is the purpose of performing a slow or static PV loop?

    _____

    _____

    _____

47. How is the inflation portion of the PV loop utilized?

    _____

    _____

    _____

48. Once the deflation point of the PV loop is identified, what happens?

    _____

    _____

49. What is the difference between a static PV loop and a quasi-static PV loop?

    _____

    _____

50. A lung recruitment maneuver provides the following information: lower inflection point (LIP) is 10 cm $H_2O$, upper inflection point on the inspiratory limb (UIPi) is 20 cm $H_2O$, and the upper inflection point on the deflation portion of the curve (UIPd) is 5 cm $H_2O$. What should the PEEP be set at and why?

_____

_____

_____

51. To avoid overdistention in the patient from the previous question, the peak inspiratory pressure (PIP) should not exceed what pressure?

_____

52. Give three examples of types of lung recruitment maneuvers.

   a. _____

   b. _____

   c. _____

53. An ARDS patient is on pressure-controlled continuous mandatory ventilation at a rate of 10 breaths/min; inspiratory-to-expiratory ratio 1:1, PC is set at 20 cm $H_2O$ above PEEP, and PEEP is 10 cm $H_2O$. Describe how manipulating the PEEP level may be used to establish an optimal PEEP level for this patient.

_____

_____

_____

_____

_____

_____

Use the following table to answer Questions 54 and 55.

| Time | 0800 | 0805 | 0810 | 0815 | 0820 | 0825 | 0830 | 0835 | 0840 | 0845 |
|------|------|------|------|------|------|------|------|------|------|------|
| PEEP (cm $H_2O$) | 0 | 5 | 10 | 15 | 20 | 25 | 30 | 35 | 40 | 35 |
| $C_s$ (mL/cm $H_2O$) | 27 | 27 | 27 | 29 | 32 | 36 | 38 | 41 | 40 | 40 |

| Time | 0850 | 0855 | 0900 | 0905 | 0910 | 0915 | 0920 | 0925 | 0930 | 0935 |
|------|------|------|------|------|------|------|------|------|------|------|
| PEEP (cm $H_2O$) | 32.5 | 30 | 27.5 | 25 | 22.5 | 20 | 17.5 | 15 | 12.5 | 10 |
| $C_s$ (mL/cm $H_2O$) | 40 | 38 | 38 | 38 | 38 | 37 | 37 | 28 | 28 | 27 |

54. At what time, PEEP level, and $C_s$ did the UIPd point occur?

_____

55. What is the appropriate PEEP setting for this patient?

_____

56. List two reasons for placing an ARDS patient in the prone position.

   a. _____

   b. _____

57. List the six mechanisms believed to improve oxygenation with prone positioning in the ARDS patient.
    a. _____
    b. _____
    c. _____
    d. _____
    e. _____
    f. _____

58. What should be the first thing done before placing a patient in the prone position?
    _____

59. What is the absolute contraindication to prone positioning?
    _____

60. Describe the two methods used to manage the ventilatory status of patients with unilateral lung disease.
    a. _____
    b. _____

## CRITICAL THINKING QUESTIONS

1. Use the following PV loop to answer Questions a through c.

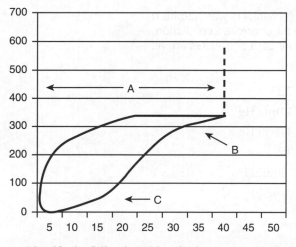

    a. Identify the following points in the pressure–volume curve.
    Point A _____
    Point B _____
    Point C _____

    b. Identify the point at which the lungs are overstretched.
    _____

    c. Identify the point that may correlate with an increase in $PaCO_2$.
    _____
    _____

2. The following volume–pressure curve was obtained from a patient receiving volume-controlled ventilation.

    a. What is the approximate PIP?
    _____

    b. What is the approximate exhaled $V_T$?
    _____

    c. By observing this volume–pressure curve, can it be determined whether the high airway pressure was caused by a decrease in the compliance or by an increase in the airway resistance?
    _____
    _____

3. A patient with ARDS and refractory hypoxemia is being ventilated in a pressure-control mode. The physician would like to perform a recruitment maneuver with increased PEEP. Can you explain the process to the physician's medical student who is asking how it works?
    _____
    _____
    _____

## CASE STUDIES

### Case Study 1

A 38-year-old patient is admitted to the emergency department and placed on volume-controlled mechanical ventilation for aspiration pneumonia. A postintubation radiograph reveals that the endotracheal tube is in proper position. There is complete opacification of the right lung. The left lung appears normal. The PIP 62 cm $H_2O$, and $P_{plat}$ 55 cm $H_2O$. The ventilator settings and ABG results are as follows:

| Mode | VC-CMV | pH | 7.43 |
|------|--------|-----|------|
| $F_1O_2$ | 1.0 | $PaCO_2$ | 38 mm Hg |
| Frequency | 20 | $P_aO_2$ | 40 mm Hg |
| $V_T$ | 800 mL | $HCO_3^-$ | 23 mEq/L |
| PEEP | 15 cm $H_2O$ | BE | 0 mEq/L |

1. What could be causing the severe hypoxemia?

_____

_____

2. What should the therapist recommend?

_____

_____

### Case Study 2

A 26-year-old male is 5 feet 6 inches tall and weighs 56.8 kg (125 lb). He was admitted for a heroin overdose and was intubated and placed on volume-controlled ventilation. Chest radiograph reveals bilateral "fluffy" infiltrates. Ventilatory data and ABGs are as follows:

| Mode | VC-CMV | pH | 7.37 |
|------|--------|-----|------|
| $F_1O_2$ | 1.0 | $PaCO_2$ | 43 mm Hg |
| Frequency | 12 | $P_aO_2$ | 44 mm Hg |
| $V_T$ | 600 mL | $S_aO_2$ | 85% |
| PEEP | 5 cm $H_2O$ | $HCO_3^-$ | 23 mEq/L |
| PIP | 55 cm $H_2O$ | BE | 0 mEq/L |
| $P_{plat}$ | 48 cm $H_2O$ | | |

1. Interpret the ABG.

_____

2. What is the significance of the $P_{plat}$?

_____

_____

3. What should the therapist recommend to treat the hypoxemia and high ventilating pressures?

_____

_____

## NBRC-STYLE QUESTIONS

1. By what mechanism does PEEP cause an increase in intracranial pressure?
   a. Cardiac output and venous return are increased.
   b. Stroke volume is decreased.
   c. There is an increase in central venous pressure.
   d. Venous return is decreased, which results in intracranial hemorrhage.

2. Which of the following is an absolute contraindication to the use of PEEP or CPAP therapy?
   a. Increased intracranial pressure
   b. Severe hyperventilation
   c. Decreased lung compliance
   d. Untreated pneumothorax or tension pneumothorax

3. A 35-year-old patient diagnosed with ARDS is receiving pressure-controlled mechanical ventilation. Based on ABG results, the PEEP is increased from 14 to 18 cm $H_2O$. Which of the following should the therapist monitor immediately after making the change?
   a. Cardiac output
   b. Pulse oximetry
   c. Hemoglobin
   d. Serum potassium

4. If the total arterial content of oxygen ($CaO_2$) is 16.94 vol%, and the cardiac output is 12.54 L/min, how much oxygen is being delivered?
   a. 1000 mL/min
   b. 2.124 L/min
   c. 3.450 L/min
   d. 3.926 L/min

5. Which of the following is the primary mechanism by which the PEEP increases $P_aO_2$ and improves the compliance?
   a. Reduction in the mean airway pressure
   b. Increase in the minute ventilation
   c. Recruitment of the collapsed alveoli
   d. Decrease in the cardiac output

6. What effect does PEEP have on both $P_aO_2$ and $PaCO_2$?
   a. Both $P_aO_2$ and $PaCO_2$ should increase.
   b. $P_aO_2$ should increase and $PaCO_2$ should decrease.
   c. Both $P_aO_2$ and $PaCO_2$ should decrease.
   d. $PaCO_2$ should remain unaffected and $P_aO_2$ should increase.

7. Which of the following is a direct lung insult that can result in ARDS?
   1. Pneumonia
   2. Aspiration
   3. Sepsis
   4. Smoke inhalation
   a. 1 only
   b. 1 and 2
   c. 1, 2, and 4
   d. 2, 3, and 4

8. Which of the following conditions is a potential complication when instituting PEEP therapy?
   1. Increase in cardiac output
   2. Barotrauma
   3. Altered cardiac function
   4. Decrease in urine output
   a. 1 only
   b. 3 and 4
   c. 1, 3 and 4
   d. 2, 3, and 4

9. What could be the most likely cause of an increased $PaCO_2$ after an increase in the level of PEEP?
   a. Tension pneumothorax
   b. Lung overdistention
   c. An increase in the compliance
   d. A decrease in the airway resistance

10. When managing a patient with ARDS receiving mechanical ventilation and PEEP, what can be done to help alleviate the problem of excessive lung water?
    a. Ventilate with large tidal volumes.
    b. Increase the amount of intravenous fluids.
    c. Patients should be placed on diuretic therapy.
    d. Keep the PIPs below 50 cm $H_2O$.

# 14 Ventilator-Associated Pneumonia

## LEARNING OBJECTIVES

*Upon completion of this chapter, the reader will be able to do the following:*

1. Define ventilator-associated pneumonia (VAP) and hospital-acquired pneumonia (HAP).
2. Differentiate between early-onset VAP and late-onset VAP and describe the overall incidence of VAP.
3. Discuss the prognosis, including morbidity and mortality rates, for patients diagnosed with VAP.
4. Identify the most common pathogenic microorganisms associated with VAP.
5. List nonpharmacological and pharmacological therapeutic interventions that have been shown to increase the risk for development of VAP.
6. Describe the sequence of events that are typically associated with the pathogenesis of VAP.
7. Discuss the advantages and disadvantages of using clinical findings versus quantitative diagnostic techniques to identify patients with VAP.
8. Briefly describe the criteria for starting empirical antibiotic therapy for patients without evidence of multidrug-resistant (MDR) infections and for those patients with risk for developing MDR infections.
9. Define de-escalation of antibiotic therapy and how it can be used to reduce the emergence of MDR pathogens.
10. Discuss how ventilator bundles can be used to prevent VAP and the emergence of MDR pathogens in the clinical setting.

**KEY TERMS CROSSWORD PUZZLE**

**Across**

1 VAP that develops later than 72 hours following tracheal intubation (two words)
3 Infection by multiple pathogenic microorganisms
5 Pathogens resistant to certain antibiotics (abbreviation)
7 A major complication of VAP
9 Assessment criteria including fever, leukocyte count, tracheal secretion characteristics, and oxygenation status
12 Guidelines for the management of adults with HAP, VAP, and health care-associated pneumonia (abbreviation)
13 Pneumonia that develops 48 hours after a patient has been placed on mechanical ventilation (abbreviation)
14 Infection acquired in the health care setting

**Down**

2 VAP that develops between 48 and 72 hours after tracheal intubation (two words)
4 Used to obtain cultures from the lower respiratory tract
6 Continuous aspiration of subglottic secretions
8 Prolonged antibiotic use for intensive care unit (ICU) patients may favor selection with resistant organisms responsible for this (two words)
10 Bronchial alveolar lavage (abbreviation)
11 Common respiratory infection seen in patients with cystic fibrosis (abbreviation)

## CHAPTER REVIEW QUESTIONS

1. VAP is most often caused by what type of infection?
   _____

2. What are the two classifications of VAP? Describe the differences.
   a. _____
   
   b. _____

3. What are some common gram-negative anaerobes isolated from nosocomial pneumonias?
   _____
   
   _____
   
   _____

4. List two common gram-positive aerobes isolated from nosocomial pneumonias?
   a. _____
   
   b. _____

5. What is the mortality rate range associated with VAP?
   _____

6. What do the guidelines for the management of patients with VAP focus on?
   _____
   
   _____
   
   _____

7. What is one of the most common nosocomial infections encountered in the ICU?
   _____

8. The incidence of VAP for all intubated patients ranges between what percentages?
   _____

9. List five causes of VAP.
   a. _____
   
   b. _____
   
   c. _____
   
   d. _____
   
   e. _____

10. List ten host-related factors that may increase the development of VAP in a patient.
    a. _____
    
    b. _____
    
    c. _____
    
    d. _____
    
    e. _____
    
    f. _____

g. _____

h. _____

i. _____

j. _____

11. What types of patients are typically at highest risk for the development of VAP?
    _____

12. Mechanically ventilated patients with chronic obstructive pulmonary disease (COPD) are susceptible to what VAP-causing pathogens?
    _____
    
    _____
    
    _____

13. Mechanically ventilated patients with cystic fibrosis are more susceptible to what VAP-causing pathogens?
    _____
    
    _____

14. VAP is a major complication of and increases the mortality rate for patients with what respiratory condition?
    _____

15. List four common risk factors for the development of MDR infections.
    a. _____
    
    b. _____
    
    c. _____
    
    d. _____

16. List six nonpharmacologic interventions that are associated with increased risk of VAP.
    a. _____
    
    b. _____
    
    c. _____
    
    d. _____
    
    e. _____
    
    f. _____

17. List four pharmacologic interventions that can lead to the development of VAP.
    a. _____
    
    b. _____
    
    c. _____
    
    d. _____

18. Describe briefly the sequence of events that leads to VAP.

_____

_____

19. What are the six clinical assessments of the Clinical Pulmonary Infection Score (CPIS) criteria?

a. _____

b. _____

c. _____

d. _____

e. _____

f. _____

20. What happens to the oropharyngeal flora of invasively ventilated, critically ill patients?

_____

21. When using all six criteria of the CPIS, what score indicates evidence of the presence of VAP?

_____

22. What procedure has been shown to significantly improve the diagnosis of VAP?

_____

23. What is the difference between clinical assessment (qualitative) and quantitative diagnosis of VAP?

_____

24. The most important nonpharmacologic prevention strategy to reduce the risk of clinicians transmitting infectious microorganisms from one patient to another is what?

_____

25. What are some ways to reduce aspiration of gastric contents?

_____

_____

_____

26. What is a common pathogen associated with percutaneous tracheostomy?

27. To lessen the risk of VAP, when should ventilator circuits be changed?

_____

28. List four pharmacologic interventions to help reduce the risk of VAP.

a. _____

b. _____

c. _____

d. _____

29. List four quantitative techniques used to diagnose VAP.

a. _____

b. _____

c. _____

d. _____

30. Successful treatment of VAP requires what two types of assessments?

a. _____

b. _____

31. What position should a ventilated patient be in to reduce the incidence of aspiration?

_____

32. Why does oral intubation pose less of a risk for VAP than nasal intubation?

_____

33. Pharmacologic and nonpharmacologic strategies to reduce the incidence of VAP are incorporated into evidence-based practices known as

_____.

## CRITICAL THINKING QUESTIONS

1. A 69-year-old male patient with a history of COPD is intubated and is receiving mechanical ventilation because of trauma sustained in a motor vehicle collision. What are some factors that put this patient at an increased risk for developing VAP and what can the therapist do to reduce this risk?

_____

_____

_____

2. Why is a patient's past medical history important when determining antibiotic therapy?

_____

## CASE STUDIES

### Case Study 1

A patient with a history of cystic fibrosis develops a fever with purulent tracheobron-chial secretions 4 days after endotracheal intubation and mechanical ventilation. The respiratory therapist suspects VAP.

1. What type of VAP is likely?

   _____

2. Considering the patient's past medical history, what is the most likely pathogen causing the pneumonia?

   _____

3. What can be done to diagnose the pathogen?

   _____

### NBRC-STYLE QUESTIONS

1. VAP is most commonly caused by which of the following?
   a. Viral infection
   b. Fungal infection
   c. Bacterial infection
   d. Acute respiratory distress syndrome
2. With regard to VAP, COPD patients are at increased risk from which of the following pathogenic organisms?
   a. *Haemophilus influenzae*
   b. *Candida albicans*
   c. *Klebsiella pneumoniae*
   d. *Pseudomonas aeruginosa*
3. Therapeutic interventions that can lead to the development of VAP include which of the following?
   a. Inappropriate antimicrobial therapy
   b. Frequent arterial blood gas analysis
   c. Noninvasive ventilation
   d. Semirecumbent positioning of the patient
4. Which of the following falls into the category of ventilator-associated event as defined by the Centers for Disease Control and Prevention?
   1. VAP
   2. Ventilator-associated condition
   3. Infection-related ventilator-associated complication
   4. Acute respiratory distress syndrome
   a. 1 and 3 only
   b. 1 and 2 only
   c. 1, 2, and 3 only
   d. 2, 3, and 4 only
5. What is the nonpharmacologic intervention most associated with VAP?
   a. Frequent changing of the ventilator circuit
   b. Use of an endotracheal tube or tracheostomy during mechanical ventilation
   c. Use of bronchoscopes
   d. Reusable ventilator probes

6. During critical illness, the shift in the normal flora of the oropharyngeal tract to gram-negative bacilli and *Staphylococcus aureus* may be due to which of the following factors?
   1. Comorbidities
   2. Malnutrition
   3. Decreased airway pH
   4. Decreased production of proteases
   a. 1 and 3 only
   b. 1 and 2 only
   c. 3 and 4 only
   d. 2 and 4 only
7. Inappropriate use of what intervention is associated with the emergence of MDR pathogens?
   a. Noninvasive positive-pressure ventilation
   b. Antibiotics
   c. Tracheostomy tubes
   d. Fiberoptic bronchoscopy
8. Which of the following refers to the process of focusing the types and duration of antibiotics used to treat VAP?
   a. Broad-spectrum antibiotic therapy
   b. Ventilator bundles
   c. Nonpharmacologic interventions
   d. Deescalating antibiotic therapy
9. What is a benefit of the use of mini bronchoalveolar lavage as a nonbronchoscopic technique?
   a. It is less expensive than bronchoscopy.
   b. It is commonly performed by a pulmonologist.
   c. Accuracy of sampling location within the lung.
   d. Direct visualization of the sampling site can be obtained.
10. Strategies to prevent VAP include:
    a. Ventilator bundles
    b. Placing all patients in strict isolation
    c. Reduce the patients receiving mechanical ventilation
    d. Limit intubations and focus patient care on the use of continuous positive airway pressure

# 15 Sedatives, Analgesics, and Paralytics

## LEARNING OBJECTIVES

*Upon completion of this chapter, the reader will be able to do the following:*

1. List the most common sedatives and analgesics used in the treatment of critically ill patients.
2. Discuss the indications, contraindications, and potential side effects associated with each of the sedatives and analgesic agents reviewed.
3. Describe the most common method for assessing the need for and level of sedation.
4. Describe the Ramsay scale.
5. Discuss the advantages and disadvantages of using benzodiazepines, neuroleptics, anesthetic agents, and opioids in the management of mechanically ventilated patients.
6. Discuss the mode of action of depolarizing and nondepolarizing paralytics.
7. Explain how the train-of-four method is used to assess the level of paralysis in critically ill patients.
8. Contrast the indications, contraindications, and potential side effects associated with using various types of neuromuscular blocking agents.
9. Recommend a medication for a mechanically ventilated patient with severe anxiety and agitation.

## KEY TERMS CROSSWORD PUZZLE

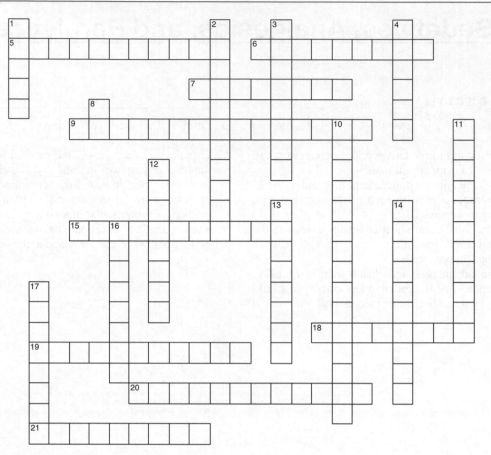

### Across

5  Type of amnesia in which the acquisition and encoding of new information that can potentially lead to memories of unpleasant experiences is prevented

6  Facilitates invasive procedures by preventing movement

7  An anesthetic agent common in the intensive care unit (ICU)

9  A depolarizing neuromuscular blocking agent

15  A graduated single-category scale that is used to assess the level of sedation (two words)

18  A benzodiazepine drug

19  Method of monitoring the depth of paralysis with an electrical current (three words)

20  An agent that causes skeletal muscle paralysis by causing a reversal of the resting membrane potential in excitable cell membranes

21  Drug of choice for sedating mechanically ventilated patients for longer than 24 hours, which generally produces only minimal effects on the cardiovascular function

### Down

1  An opioid receptor that mediates the sedative effects

2  Haloperidol is included in this category of drugs.

3  An opioid antagonist

4  Pinpoint pupils

8  An opioid receptor that is responsible for analgesia

10  Agent that inhibits the action of acetylcholine at the neuromuscular junction

11  A nondepolarizing NMBA

12  Agent that reduces anxiety and agitation and promotes sleep

13  Disorganized thought patterns and excessive, non-purposeful motor activity

14  Reverses the effects of benzodiazepines

16  A naturally occurring opioid

17  A synthetic opioid that is approximately 100 to 150 times more potent than morphine

## CHAPTER REVIEW QUESTIONS

1. What effects do sedatives have on the body?

   _____

2. Describe a clinical situation in which paralysis may be indicated during mechanical ventilation.

   _____

3. List the four types of pharmacologic agents commonly used for sedation in the ICU. Give at least one example of each.

   a. _____

   b. _____

   c. _____

   d. _____

4. List and define the four Joint Commission-defined levels of sedation.

   a. _____

   b. _____

   c. _____

   d. _____

5. What level of sedation may be necessary when a patient's breathing is asynchronous with the mechanical ventilatory mode?

   _____

6. What level of sedation is necessary during weaning from mechanical ventilation?

   _____

7. What scoring systems may be used to assess the level of sedation in adults and children?

   _____

Use the Scoring System in Table 15.1 to answer Questions 8 through 10.

### TABLE 15.1   The Ramsay Sedation Scale

| Score | Description |
| --- | --- |
| 1 | Patient is awake but anxious, agitated, and restless. |
| 2 | Patient is awake, cooperative, oriented, and tranquil. |
| 3 | Patient is semi-asleep but responds to verbal commands. |
| 4 | Patient is asleep and has a brisk response to a light glabellar tap or loud auditory stimulus. |
| 5 | Patient is asleep and has a sluggish response to a light glabellar tap or loud auditory stimulus. |
| 6 | Patient is asleep and has no response to a light glabellar tap or loud auditory stimulus. |

8. What range of scores indicates adequate sedation?

   _____

9. What score indicates the need for sedation?

   _____

10. What scores indicate oversedation of a patient?

    _____

11. Why are benzodiazepines the drugs of choice for the treatment of anxiety in critical care?

    _____
    _____

12. Explain the mode of action for benzodiazepines.

    _____
    _____
    _____
    _____

13. List three factors that can alter the intensity and duration of action of various benzodiazepines.
    a. _____
    b. _____
    c. _____

14. Describe a pathologic process that can prolong recovery from treatment with benzodiazepines.

    _____

15. Why does diazepam have a rapid onset of action?

    _____
    _____
    _____

16. How is diazepam administered in the ICU setting?

    _____
    _____

17. Acutely agitated patients are best treated with which benzodiazepine? Why?

    _____
    _____

18. How can prolonged sedation occur with midazolam?

    _____
    _____
    _____

19. Which benzodiazepine is best suited for sedating mechanically ventilated patients in the ICU for longer than 24 hours?

_____

20. You are the respiratory therapist working in the emergency department of a busy hospital. A patient is brought in, who was found unresponsive with an empty bottle of Valium near him. What medication would you suggest to reverse the drug? Are there any side effects that you would be concerned about following its administration?

_____

21. Potential side effects of continual use of lorazepam (Ativan) include the following:

a. _____

b. _____

c. _____

22. What class of drugs is routinely used to treat extremely agitated and delirious patients in the ICU?

_____

23. What is the name of the drug most often used to treat ICU delirium?

24. List three of the side effects of the drug in Question 23.

a. _____

b. _____

c. _____

25. List the hemodynamic effects of propofol.

_____

_____

26. What are the advantages and disadvantages of using propofol drug to sedate neurologic patients?

| **Disadvantages** | **Advantages** |
| --- | --- |
| _____ | _____ |
| _____ | _____ |
| _____ | _____ |
| _____ | _____ |
| _____ | _____ |
| _____ | _____ |

27. List the two opioids most commonly used in the ICU setting.

a. _____

b. _____

28. List three effects that opiates have on the body.
   a. _____
   b. _____
   c. _____

29. List ten side effects of opioids.
   a. _____
   b. _____
   c. _____
   d. _____
   e. _____
   f. _____
   g. _____
   h. _____
   i. _____
   j. _____

30. What determines the severity of the side effects of opioids?
   _____

31. Which drug can reverse the respiratory depression caused by opioids?
   _____

32. What effects does morphine have on the central nervous system?
   _____
   _____
   _____

33. How does morphine affect the gastrointestinal tract?
   _____
   _____
   _____

34. How does morphine affect the cardiovascular system?
   _____
   _____

35. Which opioid should be used for a patient who is hemodynamically unstable?
   _____

36. Increased intracranial pressure caused by traumatic brain injury may be controlled by a combination of which two drugs?
   _____

37. What is the difference between depolarizing and non-depolarizing agents?
   _____

38. List four clinical situations that may require NMBAs to be used while a patient is being mechanically ventilated.
   a. _____
   b. _____
   c. _____
   d. _____

39. What is the purpose of TOF?
   _____

40. Describe how TOF works.
   _____
   _____
   _____

41. According to the Society for Critical Care Medicine, what indicates that an adequate amount of NMBA is being administered when TOF is used?
   _____

42. What other medication is necessary when a paralytic agent is used?
   _____
   _____

43. The most widely used NMBA for facilitating endotracheal intubation is _____.

   Its onset of action and duration of action is
   _____.

44. What are the most common side effects of the drug referred to in Question 43?
   _____
   _____
   _____

45. Which nondepolarizing NMBA has the longest duration of action?
   _____

46. Which nondepolarizing NMBAs are used for intermediate duration?
   _____
   _____

47. What type of patient could experience prolonged paralysis after discontinuation of pancuronium? Why?

    _____

    _____

    _____

    _____

48. Seizures have been associated with which nondepolarizing NMBA?

    _____

49. Mast cell degranulation and histamine release, which may lead to peripheral vasodilation and hypotension, are associated with which nondepolarizing NMBA?

    _____

50. Which nondepolarizing NMBAs are ideal for patients with renal and hepatic insufficiency?

    _____

51. The nondepolarizing NMBA of choice for patients who are hemodynamically unstable, have cardiac disease, or are at risk of histamine release is

    _____.

52. List two side effects of the long-term use of NMBAs.

    a. _____

    b. _____

## CRITICAL THINKING QUESTIONS

1. When an NMBA is administered to a patient receiving ventilatory care, what ventilator alarms should be activated?

   _____

   _____

2. Which type of opioid is best suited to a patient who has asthma? Why?

   _____

   _____

   _____

   _____

## CASE STUDIES

### Case Study 1

The respiratory therapist checks on an ICU patient receiving ventilatory support with ventilator-controlled intermittent mandatory ventilation (VC-IMV). The ventilator settings are as follows: rate = 6 breaths/min, $V_T$ = 600 mL, $F_IO_2$ = 0.4, positive end-expiratory pressure = 5 cm $H_2O$. The mode was changed to VC-IMV 1 hour ago because of dyssynchrony. The patient's legs are hanging over the bed railing, and his hands are on the ventilator tubing. The high-pressure alarm is activating with every breath at a rate of 35 breaths/min. The patient is anxious and uncooperative and remains dyssynchronous with the ventilator despite adjustments made to the ventilator settings.

1. What would be the most appropriate type of medication to deliver at this time?

   _____

2. What concerns should the respiratory therapist have about the patient's ventilator settings?

   _____

   _____

   _____

## NBRC-STYLE QUESTIONS

1. Which of the following drugs can be used to reverse the effects of benzodiazepines?
   a. Pseudocholinesterase
   b. Flumazenil (Romazicon)
   c. Fentanyl citrate (Sublimaze)
   d. Naloxone (Narcan)
2. The respiratory therapist is called to the postanesthesia care unit to assist in the weaning of a postoperative patient who had a cholecystectomy. The patient is 3 hours postop and is still apneic and receiving full ventilatory support. The medication(s) that could be used to facilitate ventilator weaning is (are) which of the following?
   1. Naloxone (Narcan)
   2. Propofol (Diprivan)
   3. Midazolam (Versed)
   4. Flumazenil (Romazicon)
   a. 1 and 4 only
   b. 2 and 4 only
   c. 1 and 3 only
   d. 2 and 3 only
3. An adult patient is in pain, panicky, and fighting the ventilator. The most appropriate medication to control this patient during mechanical ventilation is which of the following?
   a. Propofol (Diprivan)
   b. Haloperidol (Haldol)
   c. Fentanyl citrate (Sublimaze)
   d. Succinylcholine (Anectine)
4. Which of the following is a fast-acting NMBA that is often used to facilitate intubation?
   a. Vecuronium (Norcuron)
   b. Pancuronium (Pavulon)
   c. Midazolam (Versed)
   d. Succinylcholine (Anectine)
5. A mechanically ventilated patient who is hemodynamically unstable needs to be placed on pressure control inverse ratio ventilation and will require paralysis. The most appropriate drug combination for this patient is which of the following?
   a. Succinylcholine chloride (Anectine) and morphine
   b. Propofol (Diprivan) and fentanyl (Sublimaze)
   c. Atracurium besylate (Tracrium) and midazolam (Versed)
   d. Cisatracurium besylate (Nimbex) and flumazenil (Romazicon)

6. A patient with which of the following Ramsay scores is most likely to wean successfully from mechanical ventilation?
   a. 1
   b. 2
   c. 4
   d. 6
7. The depth of paralysis during neuromuscular blockade may be assessed with which of the following?
   a. Ramsay scale
   b. Serum GABA levels
   c. TOF monitoring
   d. Level of sedation assessment
8. The NMBA that causes histamine release is which of the following?
   a. Atracurium
   b. Cisatracurium
   c. Vecuronium
   d. Pancuronium
9. The NMBA most appropriate for facilitating emergency intubation is which of the following?
   a. Pancuronium (Pavulon)
   b. Vecuronium (Norcuron)
   c. Atracurium (Tracrium)
   d. Succinylcholine (Anectine)
10. The NMBA that can be used in patients with renal or hepatic insufficiency without producing prolonged paralysis is which of the following?
    a. Cisatracurium (Nimbex)
    b. Vecuronium (Norcuron)
    c. Pancuronium (Pavulon)
    d. Succinylcholine (Anectine)

# 16 Extrapulmonary Effects of Mechanical Ventilation

## LEARNING OBJECTIVES

*On completion of this chapter, the reader will be able to do the following:*

1. Explain the effects of positive pressure ventilation on cardiac output and venous return to the heart.
2. Discuss the three factors that can influence cardiac output during positive pressure ventilation.
3. Explain the effects of positive pressure ventilation on gas distribution and pulmonary blood flow in the lungs.
4. Describe how positive pressure ventilation increases intracranial pressure.
5. Summarize the effects of positive pressure ventilation on renal and endocrine function.
6. Describe the effects of abnormal arterial blood gases on renal function.
7. Name five ways of assessing a patient's nutritional status.
8. Describe techniques that can be used to reduce complications associated with mechanical ventilation.

## KEY TERMS CROSSWORD PUZZLE

**Across**

4 This pressure is increased by an inflation hold (two words).
10 Gas always follows the path of _____ resistance.
12 Spontaneous inspiration increases blood flow to this structure (two words).
15 18 across plus ICP equals this (abbreviation).
18 The amount of blood flowing to the brain is determined by this (abbreviation).
19 A reduction in this decreases preload to the heart (two words).
20 Through the wall of an organ
21 Antidiuretic hormone release results in this.
22 The volume pumped out of a ventricle with one beat
24 This maneuver will increase inspiratory time (two words).
25 Inflammation of many nerves simultaneously

**Down**

1 A mechanism that maintains blood pressure (BP) in normal individuals receiving PPV
2 A function that can be altered by mechanical ventilation
3 This may decrease with the use of PPV (two words).
5 Reduction in blood flow or supply of oxygenated blood to an organ
6 The structural and functional unit of the kidney
7 Reductions in 19 across decrease this.
8 This pressure falls with spontaneous inspiration.
9 A drug used to avoid gastrointestinal bleeding
11 When an alveolus is overfilled, this capillary becomes thin
13 A reflex that is blocked by 25 across
14 Compression of the heart
16 The vein that is visible when the central venous pressure (CVP) is elevated
17 Urinary output will decrease when this capillary pressure decreases below 75 mm Hg.
23 Measuring this provides information about a patient's daily caloric requirements (abbreviation).

## CHAPTER REVIEW QUESTIONS

1. List the five bodily functions that positive pressure ventilation (PPV) can significantly alter.

   a. _____  d. _____

   b. _____  e. _____

   c. _____

2. The physiologic effects of PPV on the cardiovascular system depend on what two factors?
   _____

3. Explain how spontaneous inspiration facilitates venous return to the right heart.
   _____
   _____
   _____

4. During what part of a spontaneous breath is the right ventricular preload increased? Why?
   _____
   _____

5. During what part of a spontaneous breath is the left ventricular preload decreased? Why?
   _____
   _____
   _____

6. What will an increase in the CVP will do to the pressure gradient between the systemic veins and the right heart?
   _____

Questions 7 through 9 refer to Figure 16.1.

| Point Y1 | Point Y2 | Point Y3 |
| Pressure = 1 cm $H_2O$ | Pressure = 3 cm $H_2O$ | Pressure = 4.5 cm $H_2O$ |

| Point X1 | Point X2 | Point X3 |
| Pressure = 5 cm $H_2O$ | Pressure = 5 cm $H_2O$ | Pressure = 5 cm $H_2O$ |

A        B        C

7. Which diagram represents the largest pressure gradient?
   _____

8. Which diagram represents the smallest pressure gradient?
   _____

9. If each tube in the figure represented the inferior vena cava, the "X" points represented systemic pressure, and the "Y" points represented CVP, which diagram would have the most venous return?

10. What effect does alveolar overdistention have on the pulmonary capillaries and right ventricular afterload?

_____

_____

_____

_____

11. What conditions need to exist for the interventricular septum to move to the left during PPV?

_____

12. How can PPV cause myocardial ischemia?

_____

_____

_____

13. List the compensatory mechanisms responsible for the maintenance of systemic blood pressure during the ventilation of normal individuals.

a. _____

b. _____

c. _____

d. _____

14. List four factors that can block the body's compensatory mechanisms for maintaining the arterial blood pressure while a patient is receiving PPV.

a. _____

b. _____

c. _____

d. _____

15. How can a respiratory therapist check that normal vascular reflexes are intact when PPV is being initiated?

_____

16. Normovolemic patients may experience decreases in the cardiac output when the positive end-expiratory pressure (PEEP) levels of _____ are used.

17. List the three factors that can influence the cardiac output during PPV.

a. _____

b. _____

c. _____

18. Explain how PPV can benefit the cardiac function of a patient with left ventricular dysfunction.

_____

_____

19. What pressure exerts the most influence on the extent of harmful effects caused by PPV?

_____

20. Calculate the mean airway pressure using the following parameters: peak inspiratory pressure (PIP) 25 cm $H_2O$, $T_I$ 1 second, and respiratory rate 12 breaths/min.

_____

_____

_____

21. Add a 1-second inspiratory hold to the previous parameters from question 20 and calculate the mean airway pressure.

_____

_____

_____

22. What happens to the mean airway pressure when an inspiratory hold is added?

_____

23. Calculate the mean airway pressure using the following parameters: PIP 35 cm $H_2O$, PEEP 10 cm $H_2O$, $T_I$ 1 second, and respiratory rate 12 breaths/min. (Notice the $\Delta P$ is the same as the PIP in the previous examples.)

_____

_____

_____

_____

24. Calculate the mean airway pressure using the same parameters as in the previous example but add a 1-second inspiratory hold.

_____

_____

_____

25. What type of inspiratory flow produces uneven ventilation?

_____

26. List an inspiratory-to-expiratory ratio that is most likely to cause air trapping and significant hemodynamic complications.

_____

27. What type of $T_E$ allows for better alveolar emptying and less chance of developing intrinsic PEEP?

_____

28. The amount of mean airway pressure required to achieve a certain level of oxygenation may indicate _____.

29. List five factors that influence the mean airway pressure during mechanical ventilation.
    a. _____
    b. _____
    c. _____
    d. _____
    e. _____

30. Explain why rapid inspiratory flow rates may produce lower mean airway pressures in patients with normal conducting airways.
    _____
    _____

31. For PEEP levels to affect the cardiac output, what circumstances have to exist?
    _____
    _____
    _____

32. High levels of PEEP would not cause a decrease in the cardiac output in what circumstance?
    _____
    _____
    _____

33. What is the cerebral perfusion pressure when the ICP is 18 cm $H_2O$ and the mean systemic arterial BP is 85 cm $H_2O$?
    _____

34. How can PPV increase ICP?
    _____
    _____
    _____
    _____

35. How can an increased ICP be observed clinically?
    _____

36. What effect does hyperventilation have on cerebral vessels?
    _____

37. List three ways the renal function can be altered by PPV.
    a. _____
    b. _____
    c. _____

38. At what glomerular capillary pressure will urinary output become severely reduced?
    _____
    _____

39. What happens to the kidney function when blood flow to the outer cortex decreases and flow to the inner cortex and outer medullary tissue increases?
    _____
    _____

40. List the three hormones that are involved in fluid and electrolyte balance during PPV and what effects each of these hormones exert.
    a. _____
    b. _____
    c. _____

41. Describe the effects of abnormal arterial blood gases on the renal function.
    _____
    _____
    _____
    _____

42. What effects does PPV have on the pharmokinetics of certain drugs?
    _____
    _____
    _____

43. How can PPV and PEEP affect the liver function?
    _____
    _____
    _____
    _____

44. What causes gastric distention in patients receiving PPV, and how can it be reduced?
    _____
    _____
    _____

45. Why are medical and surgical patients subject to malnutrition during serious illness?
    _____
    _____
    _____

46. List three deleterious effects that nutritional depletion can have on mechanically ventilated patients.

    a. _____

    b. _____

    c. _____

47. What effects can overfeeding have on a mechanically ventilated patient?

    _____

    _____

    _____

48. List five ways of assessing a patient's nutritional status.

    a. _____

    b. _____

    c. _____

    d. _____

    e. _____

49. How can some of the complications associated with mechanical ventilation be reduced?

    _____

    _____

    _____

## CRITICAL THINKING QUESTIONS

1. Describe the cardiovascular effects, represented by the lettered arrows, that PPV is having on the heart in Figure 16.2.

A. _____

B. _____

C. _____

D. _____

## CASE STUDIES

### Case Study 1

A 30-year-old, 5-foot 8-inch male postoperative patient with no lung disease is in the surgical intensive care unit receiving full mechanical support with the following ventilator settings: volume-controlled continuous mandatory ventilation (VC-CMV) rate 12 breaths/min, $V_T$ 560 mL, flow rate 84 L/min, PEEP +10 cm $H_2O$, and $F_IO_2$ 0.5. His PIP is averaging around 30 cm $H_2O$ and the plateau pressure is measured at 23 cm $H_2O$.

1. Calculate this patient's mean airway pressure.

    _____

    _____

    _____

    _____

    _____

    _____

2. Analyze the patient's arterial blood gas on these ventilator settings: pH 7.38, $PCO_2$ 42 mm Hg, $PO_2$ 78 mm Hg, $S_aO_2$ 90%, and $HCO_3^-$ 23 mEq/L.

_____

_____

3. What is the most appropriate ventilator change at this time and why?

_____

_____

_____

_____

_____

## NBRC-STYLE QUESTIONS

1. What effect does the normal thoracic pump mechanism have on cardiac output (CO)?
   a. Reduces CO in normal individuals
   b. Improves CO in healthy individuals
   c. Improves CO in individuals with disease
   d. Improves CO in mechanically ventilated patients only

2. During PPV and PPV with PEEP, which of the following is true regarding the thoracic pump mechanism?
   a. CO is decreased and venous return is decreased.
   b. Left ventricular output is decreased and CO is increased.
   c. Left ventricular stroke volume is decreased and CO is decreased.
   d. Right heart venous return is increased and BP is increased.

3. The greatest reductions in venous return and cardiac output are most likely to occur during the use of which of the following ventilator modes?
   a. Continuous positive airway pressure (CPAP) 8 cm $H_2O$
   b. Intermittent mandatory volume (IMV) 10, $V_T$ 450 mL
   c. VC-CMV 12 with $V_T$ 475 mL
   d. VC-CMV 10, $V_T$ 435 mL, PEEP +6 cm $H_2O$

4. A patient's inability to compensate for diminished cardiac output during PPV will result in which of the following?
   a. Severe hemorrhage
   b. Increased BP
   c. Compromised perfusion
   d. Maintenance of normal BP

5. For which of the following reasons are patients with acute respiratory distress syndrome less likely to experience hemodynamic changes during PPV, even with high ventilatory pressures?
   a. They have elevated systemic BP.
   b. Their blood vessel walls have become too thick.
   c. Pressure is not transmitted to the pleural space.
   d. Pressure is lost in the poorly conductive airways.

6. Hazardous cardiovascular side effects in patients with severe bronchospasm are due to which of the following?
   a. Short inspiratory times
   b. Presence of auto-PEEP
   c. Elevated mean airway pressure
   d. Elevated peak inspiratory pressure

7. The pressure that has the most influence on the hemodynamic effects of PPV is which of the following?
   a. PEEP
   b. Peak pressure
   c. Plateau pressure
   d. Mean airway pressure

8. Methods of increasing the mean airway pressure include which of the following?
   1. Increasing the PEEP
   2. Increasing the total cycle time
   3. Decreasing the inspiratory time
   4. Adding an inflation hold
   a. 1 and 2 only
   b. 1 and 4 only
   c. 2 and 3 only
   d. 2 and 4 only

9. The risk of cardiovascular complications is least with the use of which of the following ventilator modes?
   a. Pressure-controlled (PC)-CMV
   b. VC-CMV with PEEP
   c. PC-IMV with pressure support
   d. CPAP with pressure support

10. The anticipated effects of PPV on the kidneys include which of the following?
    1. Diuresis
    2. Sodium retention
    3. Decreased urinary output
    4. Increased creatinine excretion
    a. 1 and 2 only
    b. 2 and 3 only
    c. 3 and 4 only
    d. 1 and 4 only

# 17 Effects of Positive Pressure Ventilation on the Pulmonary System

## LEARNING OBJECTIVES

*Upon completion of this chapter, the reader will be able to do the following:*

1. Recognize the presence of barotrauma or extraalveolar air based on patient assessment.
2. Recommend an appropriate intervention for the treatment of patients with barotrauma.
3. Evaluate findings from a patient with acute respiratory distress syndrome to establish an optimum positive end-expiratory pressure (PEEP) and ventilation strategy.
4. Identify situations in which chest wall rigidity can alter transpulmonary pressures and acceptable plateau pressures.
5. Name the types of ventilator-induced lung injury caused by opening and closing of the alveoli and overdistention of the alveoli.
6. Compare the clinical findings associated with hyperventilation and hypoventilation.
7. Recommend ventilator settings for patients demonstrating hyperventilation and hypoventilation.
8. Describe clinical laboratory findings associated with metabolic acid–base disturbances.
9. Identify a patient with air trapping.
10. Provide strategies to reduce auto-PEEP.
11. Suggest methods to reduce the work of breathing during mechanical ventilation.
12. List the possible responses to an increase in the mean airway pressure in a patient on mechanical ventilation.
13. Describe the effects of positive pressure ventilation on pulmonary gas distribution and pulmonary perfusion in relation to normal spontaneous breathing.

**KEY TERMS CROSSWORD PUZZLE**

**Across**

2 Like blebs, these focal regions in the chest wall increase risk of rupture of the lung.
5 Caused by too much volume in the alveoli
7 Occurs with overdistention of more compliant areas of the lung
12 General name for mediators released as a result of lung injury
15 Type of asynchrony caused by more than one breath type delivered by the ventilator
16 Abbreviation for lung injury at the level of the acinus
17 Described as alveolar rupture, interstitial emphysema, or perivascular and alveolar hemorrhage, which can eventually lead to death
18 Circulation of mediators cause this type of failure
19 Maneuver that causes pleural pressure to be positive
21 Asynchrony caused by inappropriate baseline settings
24 Type of trauma caused by high levels of pressure
28 One type of mediator released as a result of lung injury
29 Touching subcutaneous emphysema feels like this
30 Closing of lung units

**Down**

1 Asynchrony caused by inadequate gas speed
3 Atelectasis caused by high oxygen concentration
4 Asynchrony caused by dual control modes of ventilation (two words)
6 Inadequate alveolar ventilation
8 The sign indicative of a tension pneumothorax on chest radiograph (two words)
9 Type of hyperinflation caused by failure of lung volume to return to passive functional residual capacity
10 Asynchrony caused by inappropriate sensitivity settings
11 Caused by release of inflammatory mediators from the lungs
13 A pneumothorax causes this to shift
14 Opening of lung units
19 Abbreviation for lung injury as a consequence of mechanical ventilation
20 Asynchrony may cause this type of chest-abdominal movement.
22 Vascular area that hemorrhages due to alveolar trauma
23 This area of the lungs receives most blood flow in the supine position.
25 Another name for auto-PEEP or intrinsic PEEP
26 Abbreviation for diaphragm's electrical activity
27 Asynchrony caused by a very long inspiratory time

## CHAPTER REVIEW QUESTIONS

1. Define *volutrauma* and *biotrauma*.

2. Briefly describe the difference between ventilator-induced lung injury and ventilator-associated lung injury.

3. List five conditions that can predispose a patient to barotrauma while he or she is being mechanically ventilated.

   a.

   b.

   c.

   d.

   e.

4. During patient ventilator system checks, the respiratory therapist notes the right lateral side of the patient's neck and face appear puffy. These areas feel crepitant to the touch; however, no distress is observed in the patient. What is the most likely cause of this problem?

5. What is likely the cause of a sudden onset of increased peak airway pressures and hyper-resonance in a patient receiving mechanical ventilation?

6. What is the treatment for a tension pneumothorax?

7. When a mechanically ventilated patient develops a tension pneumothorax, how should he or she be ventilated until the appropriate treatment can begin?

8. List four clinical signs of a tension pneumothorax.

   a.

   b.

   c.

   d.

9. How would a chest radiograph of a patient with a tension pneumothorax look?

10. What is the term used to describe air dissecting into the retroperitoneal space?

11. What is the minimum transpulmonary pressure that has been associated with lung injury in animals?

12. List three examples of clinical situations where lung injury can occur from a high transpulmonary pressure.

    a.

    b.

    c.

13. Describe how volutrauma occurs.

14. What are the three primary types of lung injury that can occur with the repeated opening and closing of the lung units? Briefly explain each.

    a.

    b.

    c.

15. Explain shear stress and how it can lead to edema formation.

16. Define atelectrauma and give a clinical situation that puts a ventilated patient at risk of developing it.

_____

_____

_____

17. List two chemical mediators that are released when the alveolar epithelial cells are overstretched.

    a. _____

    b. _____

18. Describe how multiorgan failure develops in a patient receiving mechanical ventilation.

_____

_____

_____

_____

19. How can multiorgan failure be avoided during mechanical ventilation?

_____

_____

_____

20. In what areas of the lung are ventilation and perfusion best matched during spontaneous ventilation in the supine position?

_____

_____

21. Describe how ventilation and perfusion are altered during PPV in a patient who is sedated and paralyzed.

_____

_____

_____

22. How can the changes in gas distribution during mechanical ventilation be minimized?

23. How can PPV increase the dead space?

_____

_____

_____

24. Why would the use of high volumes during PPV and PEEP cause an increase in pulmonary shunting?

_____

_____

_____

_____

25. How can mechanical ventilation cause an increase in pulmonary vascular resistance?

_____

_____

_____

26. Explain how hypoventilation can lead to cardiac dysrhythmias.

_____

27. What type of patient may benefit from permissive hypercapnia?

_____

28. List four reasons for patient-induced hyperventilation.

    a. _____

    b. _____

    c. _____

    d. _____

29. What acid–base disturbance can cause a right shift in the oxygen dissociation curve?

_____

30. Describe two clinical implications of prolonged ventilator-induced hyperventilation?

    a. _____

    _____

    b. _____

    _____

31. What happens to the cerebrospinal fluid during prolonged hyperventilation during mechanical ventilation?

_____

_____

_____

_____

32. When is the administration of intravenous bicarbonate indicated?

_____

_____

33. List four causes of metabolic alkalosis in the clinical setting.

a. _____

b. _____

c. _____

d. _____

34. What can cause auto-PEEP without dynamic hyperinflation?

_____

_____

35. Describe how ventilator-induced auto-PEEP can be created.

_____

_____

_____

_____

_____

36. What patient factors increase the risk of auto-PEEP?

_____

_____

_____

37. On the graph below, draw a flow–time curve for (VC-CMV), showing a "normal" exhalation and one exhibiting auto-PEEP.

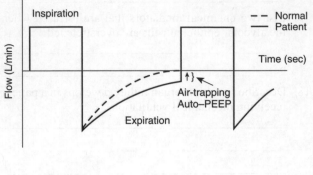

_____

_____

38. What technique is used to detect the presence of auto-PEEP?

_____

39. How many time constants are necessary for the lungs to empty 98% of the inspired volume?

_____

40. Define dynamic hyperinflation.

_____

41. What effects can the presence of auto-PEEP have on ventilator function?

_____

_____

_____

_____

_____

42. Calculate the static compliance for the following situation: $V_T$ 525 mL, peak inspiratory pressure (PIP) 43 cm $H_2O$, $P_{plat}$ 30 cm $H_2O$, set PEEP 12 cm $H_2O$, auto-PEEP 5 cm $H_2O$.

   _____

   _____

   _____

   _____

43. List four strategies that can be used to decrease the auto-PEEP when the patient is receiving full ventilatory support.

   a. _____

   b. _____

   c. _____

   d. _____

44. List four modes of ventilation that may be used to decrease the auto-PEEP in a patient who is intubated and has spontaneous breathing efforts.

   a. _____

   b. _____

   c. _____

   d. _____

45. When does pulmonary oxygen toxicity become a problem in adults and premature infants?

   _____

   _____

   _____

46. If an $F_1O_2$ of greater than _____ is required, PEEP should be used. List four ways to assess pulmonary changes associated with oxygen toxicity.

   a. _____

   b. _____

   c. _____

   d. _____

47. What are the lower limit targets for oxygenation for patients receiving mechanical ventilation?

   _____

48. What can the use of low tidal volumes with oxygen concentrations greater than 70% may lead?

   _____

49. What is the normal inspiratory WOB?

   _____

50. When is inspiratory WOB considered high?

   _____

51. What are some signs that a patient has an increased WOB?

   _____

52. Calculate the estimated WOB for a patient receiving mechanical ventilation with the following data: PIP = 45 cm $H_2O$, $P_{plat}$ = 33 cm $H_2O$, and $V_T$ = 475 mL.

   _____

   _____

   _____

   _____

53. List four basic strategies for minimizing a patient's WOB.

   a. _____

   b. _____

   c. _____

   d. _____

54. List four signs of patient–ventilator asynchrony.

   a. _____

   b. _____

   c. _____

   d. _____

55. Define trigger asynchrony and describe a method to avoid it.

_____

_____

_____

56. How can auto-PEEP cause trigger asynchrony?

_____

_____

_____

57. What should the initial flow be set at when using volume ventilation with a constant flow?

_____

58. What type of breaths may provide more synchrony for a patient with high flow demands and why?

_____

_____

_____

59. What adjustment can be made during pressure-targeted ventilation to lessen the rapid rise of flow when a breath begins?

_____

_____

60. What is cycle asynchrony and under what conditions can it occur?

_____

_____

_____

61. What strategies may be used to eliminate cycle asynchrony during mechanical ventilation with full support and spontaneous ventilation?

_____

_____

_____

62. What mode of ventilation delivers varying breath types, which may result in mode asynchrony?

63. When does PEEP asynchrony occur?

_____

_____

64. How can closed-loop ventilation lead to asynchrony?

_____

_____

_____

65. List five potential mechanical failures that can occur during mechanical ventilation.
    a. _____
    b. _____
    c. _____
    d. _____
    e. _____

66. List seven potential mechanical failures that can occur with mechanical ventilation.
    a. _____
    b. _____
    c. _____
    d. _____
    e. _____
    f. _____
    g. _____

67. What hazards are associated with the use of both heat moisture exchangers and heated humidifiers?

_____

_____

_____

## CRITICAL THINKING QUESTIONS

Questions 1 and 2 refer to the figure below.

1. What problem is shown in this pressure–time curve?

   _____

   _____

2. What change can be made to the ventilator settings to alleviate this problem?

   _____

   _____

Questions 3 and 4 refer to the figure below.

3. What problem is shown in this pressure–time curve?

   _____

   _____

4. What change can be made to the ventilator settings to alleviate this problem?

   _____

   _____

5. Which of the following patients will be more likely to develop auto-PEEP due to dynamic hyperinflation with a set rate of 12 breaths/min? Why?

   Patient #1: airway resistance = 25 cm $H_2O$/L/s and static compliance = 50 mL/cm $H_2O$

   Patient #2: airway resistance = 6 cm $H_2O$/L/s and static compliance = 25 mL/cm $H_2O$

   _____

   _____

   _____

   _____

## CASE STUDIES

### Case Study 1

A patient 4 days post single-lung transplant is being mechanically ventilated. The remaining lung is fibrotic on the chest radiograph and the transplanted lung is hyperinflated. The patient is unresponsive, cyanotic, and hypotensive. Her ideal body weight is 135 pounds. She is being ventilated with VC-CMV, and the flow sheet for the past few hours shows the following:

| Time | Set Rate | Set $V_T$ | Flow | PIP | $F_IO_2$ | PEEP | pH | $PCO_2$ | $PO_2$ |
|------|----------|-----------|------|-----|----------|------|------|---------|--------|
| 0800 | 20 | 300 | 60 | 52 | 0.7 | 0 | 7.18 | 86 | 275 |
| 1000 | 22 | 300 | 60 | 50 | 1.0 | 0 | 7.15 | 94 | 504 |
| 1200 | 24 | 300 | 60 | 55 | 1.0 | 0 | 7.14 | 95 | 95 |
| 1400 | 40 | 320 | 60 | 60 | 1.0 | 0 | 7.06 | 110 | 125 |

The $P_{plat}$ at 1400 hours was 38 cm $H_2O$.

1. What is the most apparent problem in this patient's ventilator course?

_____

_____

_____

2. What is the most likely cause of this problem?

_____

_____

_____

_____

3. What complications is this patient at risk of developing?

_____

_____

_____

_____

4. What should be the first change made to this patient's ventilator parameters?

_____

_____

### Case Study 2

A 65-year-old, 5-foot 10-inch male patient with chronic obstructive pulmonary disease (COPD) was intubated 3 days ago and is being mechanically ventilated with VC-CMV rate 14 breaths/min, $V_T$ 550 mL, $F_IO_2$ 0.3, and PEEP +3 cm $H_2O$. This patient's baseline room air arterial blood gas (ABG) is pH 7.37, $P_aCO_2$ 57 mm Hg, $P_aO_2$ 54 mm Hg, $S_aO_2$ 90%, and $HCO_3^-$ 30 mEq/L. The ABGs on the current ventilator setting are pH 7.41, $PaCO_2$ 41 mm Hg, $P_aO_2$ 70 mm Hg, $S_aO_2$ 94%, and $HCO_3^-$ 25 mEq/L. The patient is placed on volume-controlled intermittent mandatory ventilation (VC-IMV) to begin the weaning process and the mandatory rate is reduced to 6 breaths/min.

One hour after this change, the respiratory therapist is called to the patient's room because the high respiratory rate alarm is sounding. The patient is diaphoretic, anxious, tachycardic, and is using accessory muscles.

1. What is the most likely cause of this patient's failure to wean?

_____

_____

2. What could the respiratory therapist do to alleviate this problem?

_____

_____

_____

_____

3. After 48 hours, the volume-controlled intermittent mandatory ventilation (VC-IMV) is switched to pressure-support ventilation 10 cm $H_2O$. The respiratory therapist observes the pressure–time scalar shown below. What is causing the spike at the end of the wave?

_____

_____

4. How can the problem be alleviated?

_____

## Case Study 3

A 33 year-old man was endotracheal intubated for 3 hours for a surgical procedure. He was extubated after 1 day of mechanical ventilation. Thirty minutes after extubation, the nurse calls you and states he is experiencing shortness of breath. When you enter his room, you can hear stridor.

1. What is stridor?

2. What is the likely cause of stridor in this patient?

3. How would you begin assessment on this patient?

4. How would you treat him to alleviate the problem?

### NBRC-STYLE QUESTIONS

1. The major hazard(s) of oxygen therapy in association with mechanical ventilation include (s) which of the following?
   1. Tachycardia
   2. Absorption atelectasis
   3. Oxygen-induced bradypnea
   4. Pulmonary oxygen toxicity
   a. 3 only
   b. 1 and 2 only
   c. 2 and 4 only
   d. 1, 3, and 4 only

2. Auto-PEEP should be suspected during which of the following observations?
   a. There is a prolonged postexpiratory pause.
   b. The patient coughs severely when suctioned.
   c. Expiration is continuous up to the next inspiration.
   d. The IMV mandatory rate is set at 10 breaths/min.

3. The lung capacity that increases when auto-PEEP is present is which of the following?
   a. Vital capacity
   b. Inspiratory capacity
   c. Total lung capacity
   d. Functional residual capacity

4. Iatrogenic hyperventilation of a patient with a diagnosis of COPD may lead to which of the following consequences?
   1. Tetany
   2. Air trapping
   3. Cerebral edema
   4. Hypokalemia
   a. 2 only
   b. 1 and 3 only
   c. 2 and 4 only
   d. 1, 2, and 4 only

5. A patient who has been mechanically ventilated for 7 days has recently developed subcutaneous emphysema. Further assessment reveals cyanosis, signs of dyspnea, and a markedly elevated PIP. This patient is most likely experiencing which of the following?
   a. Pneumothorax
   b. Pneumoperitoneum
   c. Increased compliance
   d. Pneumomediastinum

6. The risk of volutrauma is increased for mechanically ventilated patients who exhibit which of the following?
   a. Increased PTA
   b. Decreased PA
   c. Increased PL
   d. Decreased $P_{AO}$

7. The amount of bicarbonate replacement given to a patient with severe metabolic acidosis, who weighs 145 pounds and has a base deficit of 10, should be which of the following?
   a. 55 mEq
   b. 110 mEq
   c. 220 mEq
   d. 242 mEq

8. Failure to recognize a patient's trigger efforts is known as which of the following?
   a. Mode asynchrony
   b. Flow asynchrony
   c. Trigger asynchrony
   d. Closed-loop ventilation asynchrony

9. An increase in a patient's assist rate followed by a rise in the PIP and a drop in the exhaled tidal volume is most often associated with which of the following?
   a. Auto-PEEP
   b. Mode asynchrony
   c. PEEP asynchrony
   d. Subcutaneous emphysema

10. The presence of fine, late inspiratory crackles may reflect which of the following lung injuries?
    1. Biotrauma
    2. Shear stress
    3. Surfactant alteration
    4. Subcutaneous emphysema
    a. 1 and 2 only
    b. 2 and 3 only
    c. 1 and 4 only
    d. 3 and 4 only

# 18 Troubleshooting and Problem Solving

## LEARNING OBJECTIVES

*On completion of this chapter, the reader will be able to do the following:*

1. Identify various types of technical problems encountered during mechanical ventilation of critically ill patients and describe the steps that can be used to protect a patient when problems occur.
2. Name at least two possible causes for each of the following alarm situations: Low-pressure alarm, high-pressure alarm, low-PEEP/CPAP alarms, apnea alarm, low or high tidal volume alarm, low or high minute volume alarm, low or high respiratory rate alarm, low or high $F_IO_2$ alarm, low-source gas pressure or power input alarm, ventilator inoperative alarm, and technical error message.
3. Determine the cause of a problem using ventilator graphics from a patient–ventilator system.
4. Assess a patient on mechanical ventilation, who is experiencing sudden dyspnea, and identify the cause of the problem.
5. Describe the signs and symptoms associated with patient–ventilator asynchrony.
6. Explain the correct procedure for determining whether a problem originates with the patient or the ventilator during patient–ventilator asynchrony.
7. List four ways the addition of a nebulizer powered by an external source gas can affect ventilator function.
8. Recognize abnormalities in ventilator graphics and patient response in the event of inadequate gas flow delivery to a patient.
9. Identify the causes and potential problems related to electrolyte imbalances and their causes.
10. Recognize the signs and symptoms of a respiratory infection.
11. Identify a problem associated with an artificial airway or a mask used for noninvasive positive pressure ventilation.
12. Recognize the presence of auto-PEEP using ventilator graphics.
13. Suggest appropriate interventions for a patient who has experienced a right main-stem intubation and for a patient with a pneumothorax using physical assessment data.
14. Describe the potential problems associated with using a heated humidification system during mechanical ventilation.
15. Use a ventilator flow–volume loop to assess a patient's response to bronchodilator therapy.
16. Make recommendations about ventilator parameters for a patient with acute respiratory distress syndrome.
17. Recommend adjustment of flow-cycle criteria during pressure support ventilation based on ventilator graphics.

## KEY TERMS CROSSWORD PUZZLE

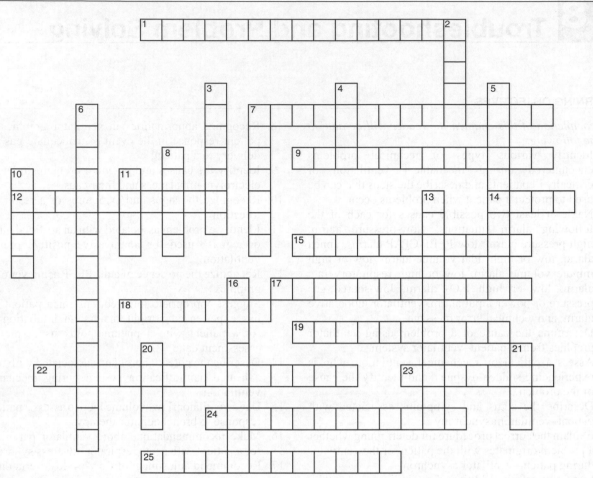

### Across

1 The type of interference caused by a cell phone
7 Fluid in the lungs (two words)
9 A life-threatening cause of severe patient distress seen in patients receiving positive-pressure ventilation
12 The artery whose wall may be eroded and can rupture within 3 weeks after a tracheostomy
14 Continuous suction endotracheal tube (abbreviation)
15 An indicator of cardiopulmonary distress
18 Waveform _____ is caused by oscillation of air in the patient–ventilator circuit at the beginning of inspiration
19 Without synchrony
22 Identification and resolution of technical malfunctions in the patient–ventilator system
23 Abnormal accumulation of edematous fluid within the peritoneal cavity
24 Smooth muscle contraction in the lungs
25 A type of therapy that breaks up blood clots

### Down

2 Active exhalation during pressure-support ventilation is a common cause of this type of dyssynchrony
3 A situation in which one finds discord or in which one is uncomfortable and does not have an immediate solution
4 This type of dyssynchrony occurs when more than one breath type is delivered
5 Inward protrusion of intercostal spaces
6 Blood clot in the lungs (two words)
7 The person attached to the ventilator
8 An alert for a clinician; it can be visual or audible.
10 The bronchus that an endotracheal tube can most easily slip into
11 An unintentional bend in the endotracheal tube
13 Especially profuse perspiration
16 Radiograph of blood vessels
20 The type of dyssynchrony that occurs when gas speed is inadequate
21 A hole in an endotracheal tube cuff may cause this

**CHAPTER REVIEW QUESTIONS**

1. Define the term *problem*.
   _____
   _____

2. Define *troubleshooting* in the context of mechanical ventilation.
   _____
   _____
   _____

3. When responding to an activated ventilator alarm, what is the respiratory therapist's first priority?
   _____
   _____

4. What assessments must be made following response to an activated ventilator alarm?
   _____
   _____
   _____

5. If a serious ventilatory problem is detected, what should the respiratory therapist do?
   _____
   _____

6. List the advantages and disadvantages of manually ventilating a patient when a problem with the ventilator is detected.
   _____
   _____
   _____
   _____
   _____

7. List five physical signs of distress that a patient receiving mechanical ventilation might exhibit.
   a. _____
   b. _____
   c. _____
   d. _____
   e. _____

8. What equipment, techniques, or data can be used to help identify the cause of a patient's sudden distress while being mechanically ventilated?
   _____
   _____
   _____

9. List six patient-related causes of sudden respiratory distress that originate within the patient's lungs.
   a. _____
   b. _____
   c. _____
   d. _____
   e. _____
   f. _____

10. List six nonpulmonary patient-related causes of sudden respiratory distress.
    a. _____
    b. _____
    c. _____
    d. _____
    e. _____
    f. _____

11. Aside from patient–ventilator asynchrony, what ventilator-related issues can cause sudden respiratory distress in patients?
    _____

12. How should the respiratory therapist distinguish between severe distress caused by a ventilator-related problem or a or patient-related problem?
    _____
    _____
    _____

13. Describe the seven steps needed to manage sudden severe distress in a ventilator-supported patient.
    a. _____
    b. _____
    c. _____
    d. _____
    e. _____
    f. _____
    g. _____

14. An oral endotracheal tube should be approximately at what mark for men and for women? What are the appropriate ranges for each?
    _____
    _____

15. What steps should be taken if a suction catheter cannot be passed down the endotracheal tube of a patient in severe respiratory distress (patient is not biting the tube)?

_____

_____

16. What clinical manifestation should a respiratory therapist look for when a tension pneumothorax is suspected during positive-pressure ventilation?

_____

_____

17. If a tension pneumothorax is strongly suspected and cardiopulmonary arrest is imminent, what action should be taken?

_____

_____

18. What signs suggest that a patient is experiencing bronchospasm while receiving mechanical ventilation?

_____

_____

_____

19. How can problems due to secretions be minimized during mechanical ventilation?

_____

_____

_____

20. What is the difference in onset between cardiogenic and noncardiogenic pulmonary edema?

_____

_____

_____

21. How does auto-PEEP affect the flow–time scalar and the flow–volume loop?

_____

_____

22. List three conditions that may stimulate output of the respiratory center.
   a. _____
   b. _____
   c. _____

23. Describe how the presence of abdominal distention can cause atelectasis, ventilation/perfusion abnormalities, and hypoxemia?

_____

_____

_____

24. The rapid onset of hypoxemia, tachycardia, tachypnea, and hypertension, along with a decrease in end-tidal $CO_2$, is indicative of what type of patient problem? How can this problem be confirmed and treated?

_____

_____

_____

25. List four sources of leaks in the patient–ventilator system.
   a. _____
   b. _____
   c. _____
   d. _____

26. List four common causes of a low-pressure alarm situation.
   a. _____
   b. _____
   c. _____
   d. _____

27. List nine common causes of a high-pressure alarm situation.
   a. _____
   b. _____
   c. _____
   d. _____
   e. _____
   f. _____
   g. _____
   h. _____
   i. _____

28. If the peak inspiratory pressure (PIP) is 30 cm $H_2O$, what should the low- and high-pressure alarms be set at?

_____

_____

29. Name two conditions that would trigger a low PEEP/CPAP alarm.

    a. _____

    b. _____

30. List five potential causes for triggering an apnea alarm.

    a. _____

    b. _____

    c. _____

    d. _____

    e. _____

31. List two potential causes for triggering a low-source gas pressure alarm.

    a. _____

    b. _____

32. List two potential causes for a power-input alarm.

    a. _____

    b. _____

33. What is the most likely cause of a "ventilator inoperative" alarm?

    _____

    _____

34. Describe the alarm situations and ventilator graphics that a leak in the patient–ventilator system would cause.

    _____

    _____

    _____

    _____

35. What types of graphics will allow the respiratory therapist to detect inadequate flow?

    _____

    _____

    _____

36. What is the phenomenon caused by the oscillation of air in the patient–ventilator circuit and at the upper airway at the beginning of inspiration?

    _____

37. What can be done to alleviate the problem caused by the phenomenon in Question 36?

    _____

    _____

38. List three problems that may cause the expiratory portion of the volume–time curve to go below baseline.

    a. _____

    b. _____

    c. _____

39. How does an externally powered nebulizer affect ventilator function?

    _____

    _____

    _____

    _____

40. A leak in the endotracheal tube cuff will cause which alarms to be activated?

    _____

    _____

41. Compare the findings from a right mainstem intubation and from a left and right tension pneumothorax by completing the following chart.

| Clinical Findings | Right Mainstem Intubation | Left-Sided Pneumothorax | Right-Sided Pneumothorax |
|---|---|---|---|
| PIP | | | |
| $P_{plat}$ | | | |
| Breath sounds | | | |
| Chest movement | | | |
| Percussion | | | |
| Tracheal shift | | | |

42. During mechanical ventilation with pressure controlled-continuous mandatory ventilation (PC-CMV), the low tidal volume alarm becomes activated on every breath; there is no leak in the system. What could be the cause of this alarm?

_____

_____

43. What situations can cause the inspiratory-to-expiratory ratio indicator and alarm to be activated?

_____

_____

_____

44. A respiratory therapist responding to a ventilator alarm finds that the high respiratory rate alarm is activated. The ventilator is set to a volume-controlled continuous mandatory ventilation (VC-CMV) rate of 12. What are some possible reasons for this activated alarm?

_____

_____

_____

## CRITICAL THINKING QUESTIONS

Questions 1 through 4 refer to the following scenario.

You are the respiratory therapist who responds to a sounding ventilator alarm. The patient has been receiving mechanical ventilation for the past 3 days, following an exacerbation of congestive heart failure and pneumonia. She has been unresponsive to verbal stimuli during this period. Her ventilator settings are VC-CMV, set rate 12 breaths/min, tidal volume 475 mL, $F_IO_2$ 0.5, and PEEP +5 cm $H_2O$. The PIP has been averaging 28 cm $H_2O$, and the $P_{plat}$ about 21 cm $H_2O$. As you approach the patient, you note that the alarm panel indicates a high-pressure condition, along with a low exhaled tidal volume and low exhaled minute volume. The patient's high-pressure alarm threshold is set at 40 cm $H_2O$ and the returned volume is 175 mL.

1. What action should the respiratory therapist take at this time?

_____

_____

_____

2. Name three conditions that could cause this situation.
   a. _____
   b. _____
   c. _____

3. Describe the best course of action to remedy each of the three conditions mentioned in the previous answer.
   a. _____
   b. _____
   c. _____

4. Why are the low exhaled tidal volume and low exhaled minute volume active along with the high-pressure alarm?

_____

_____

_____

_____

Questions 5 and 6 refer to the following scenario.

A patient recently weaned from full ventilatory support has just been switched to CPAP +10 cm $H_2O$ with pressure support of 25 cm $H_2O$. After a few spontaneous breaths on the CPAP with pressure support, the patient developed respiratory distress. The patient does not seem to be able to trigger the pressure-supported breaths, and the ventilator's apnea alarm has been activated.

5. Explain two possible causes for this patient's respiratory distress.
   a. _____
   b. _____

6. What actions could correct these possible causes?
   a. _____
   b. _____

## CASE STUDIES

### Case Study 1

1. The flow–volume loop shown in the figure below is for a patient receiving mechanical ventilation. What type of problem is demonstrated in this flow–volume loop?

2. What can be done to solve this problem?

### Case Study 2

A 42-year-old male had surgery to repair a crushed hip and femur fractures that occurred in a motor vehicle crash. Five hours after surgery, the patient continues to receive positive-pressure ventilation. Until now, the patient's condition has been stable, but he has been unconscious. At 1810 hours, a sudden change in the patient's vital signs has brought the respiratory therapist to the patient's bedside. The pulse oximetry reading has dropped from 96 to 87%, and the blood pressure (BP) has risen from 136/82 to 160/100 mm Hg. The following table shows the last patient–ventilator checks.

| Date | 5/29 | 5/29 | 5/29 | 5/29 |
|---|---|---|---|---|
| Time | 1400 | 1610 | 1750 | 1810 |
| Mode | PC-CMV | PC-CMV | PC-CMV | PC-CMV |
| Set rate | 12 | 12 | 12 | 12 |
| Total rate | 12 | 12 | 20 | 25 |
| Volume with set PIP | 620 mL | 628 mL | 625 mL | 615 mL |
| $T_I$ | 1 second | 1 second | 1 second | 1 second |
| Waveform | Square | Square | Square | Square |
| PIP (cm $H_2O$) | 30 | 28 | 32 | 33 |
| $P_{plat}$ (cm $H_2O$) | 23 | 21 | 22 | 20 |
| PEEP (cm $H_2O$) | 5 | 5 | 5 | ↑ 8 |

| Date | 5/29 | 5/29 | 5/29 | 5/29 |
|---|---|---|---|---|
| $F_IO_2$ | 0.4 | 0.4 | 0.4 | ↑ 0.6 |
| Breath sounds | Bilateral clear | Bilateral clear | Bilateral clear | Bilateral clear |
| BP (mm Hg) | 136/82 | 132/80 | 155/88 | 160/100 |
| Heart rate (BPM) | 96 | 94 | 125 | 128 |
| $SpO_2$ | 96% | 96% | 96% | 87% |
| $P_{ET}CO_2$ (mm Hg) | 36 | 36 | 34 | 26 |
| Arterial blood gases Ph | 7.43 | — | — | 7.47 |
| $PaCO_2$ (mm Hg) | 39 | — | — | 30 |
| $P_aO_2$ (mm Hg) | 98 | — | — | 78 |

1. The patient is now in obvious respiratory distress. What action should the respiratory therapist take at this time?

   _____

   _____

2. Nothing that is done seems to relieve this patient's respiratory distress. What is the most likely cause of this problem?

   _____

   _____

## Case Study 3

A 62-year-old woman is receiving ventilatory support with volume ventilation. She had abdominal surgery 10 hours ago. She has no history of smoking. Over the past few hours, the following patient information was gathered.

| Time | 0700 | 0900 | 1000 |
|---|---|---|---|
| Volume | 450 mL | 450 mL | 450 mL |
| PIP | 18 cm $H_2O$ | 24 cm $H_2O$ | 27 cm $H_2O$ |
| $P_{plat}$ | 13 cm $H_2O$ | 12 cm $H_2O$ | 14 cm $H_2O$ |

1. What is the most likely cause of the increase in PIP between 7 and 10 AM?

   _____

   _____

2. List some of the problems that can cause this type of increase in PIP.

   _____

   _____

3. What actions should the respiratory therapist take to determine the source of this patient's problem?

   _____

   _____

**NBRC-STYLE QUESTIONS**

1. During pressure-control ventilation, the alarm that identifies worsening lung compliance is which of the following?
   a. Low PEEP/CPAP
   b. High respiratory rate
   c. Low $V_T$
   d. High PIP
2. Identify the problem in the following flow–time scalar.

   a. Auto-PEEP
   b. Excessively prolonged $T_E$
   c. Inadequate $T_I$
   d. Increased airway resistance
3. Which of the following may solve the problem represented in the pressure–time scalar in below?

   a. Changing the flow waveform
   b. Increasing the pressure sensitivity
   c. Increasing the inspiratory rise time
   d. Increasing the peak pressure
4. The problem indicated in the following flow–volume loop is which of the following?

   a. Increase in the airway resistance
   b. Active exhalation against inspiration
   c. Leak in the patient–ventilator system
   d. Auto-PEEP

5. The problem indicated in the pressure–volume loop below, obtained during VC-CMV, can be solved by which of the following?

1. Suctioning of the endotracheal tube
2. Switching to PC-CMV
3. Lowering the $V_T$ in VC-CMV
4. Administering a bronchodilator
a. 1 and 2
b. 2 and 3
c. 3 and 4
d. 1 and 4

6. The problem that could cause the pressure–time scalar is which of the following?

1. Bronchoconstriction
2. High airway resistance
3. Alveolar overdistention
4. Decreased lung compliance
a. 1 and 2
b. 2 and 3
c. 3 and 4
d. 1 and 4

7. The respiratory therapist is assessing a mechanically ventilated patient who has developed sudden respiratory distress. The respiratory therapist notes that the 15-mm endotracheal tube adapter is at the level of the patient's teeth. The suspected airway problem is which of the following?
a. Cuff rupture or leakage
b. Rupture of the innominate artery
c. Patient biting the endotracheal tube
d. The endotracheal tube has slipped into the right mainstem bronchus

8. The respiratory therapist is unable to pass a suction catheter into a patient's endotracheal tube or to ventilate the patient manually with a resuscitator bag. Deflation of the cuff does not relieve the patient's distress. The most appropriate action is which of the following?
a. Reinflate the cuff and attempt ventilation again.
b. Remove the endotracheal tube and provide bag-mask ventilation.
c. Keep the cuff inflated and attempt ventilation again with 100% oxygen.
d. Deflate the cuff, suction the upper airway, and provide bag-mask ventilation.

9. What should the respiratory therapist check first when a low-pressure alarm is activated on a ventilator?
   a. Apnea parameters
   b. Patient connection
   c. 50 psi gas source
   d. Ventilator electronics

10. What problem must be present to cause simultaneous activation of the low-pressure, low-volume, and low minute ventilation alarms?
    a. Inadequate flow setting
    b. Ventilator dyssynchrony
    c. Patient–ventilator system leak
    d. Inappropriate trigger sensitivity

# 19 Basic Concepts of Noninvasive Positive Pressure Ventilation

## LEARNING OBJECTIVES

*Upon completion of this chapter, the reader will be able to do the following:*

1. Define noninvasive ventilation and discuss the three basic noninvasive techniques.
2. Discuss the clinical and physiological benefits of noninvasive positive pressure ventilation (NIV).
3. Identify the selection and exclusion criteria for NIV application in the acute and chronic care settings.
4. Compare the types of ventilators used for noninvasive ventilation.
5. Explain the importance of humidification during NIV application.
6. Describe the factors that will influence the fractional inspired oxygen concentration ($FIO_2$) from a portable pressure-targeted ventilator.
7. Identify the possible causes of rebreathing $CO_2$ during NIV administration from a portable pressure-targeted ventilator.
8. Compare the advantages and disadvantages of the various types of interfaces for the application of NIV.
9. List the steps used in the initiation of NIV.
10. Discuss several factors that affect the delivery of aerosols during NIV.
11. Identify several indicators of success for patients on NIV.
12. Make recommendations for ventilator changes based on observation of the patient's respiratory status, acid–base status, or oxygenation status.
13. Recognize the potential complications of NIV.
14. Provide optional solutions to complications of NIV.
15. Describe two basic approaches to weaning the patient from NIV.

**KEY TERMS CROSSWORD PUZZLE**

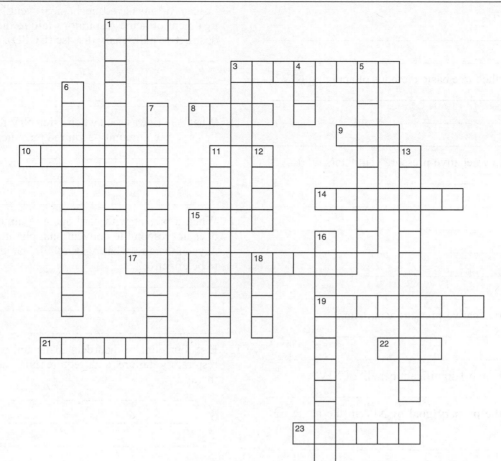

### Across

1   First-choice therapy for the treatment of obstructive sleep apnea (OSA)
3   Type of ventilator used during the polio epidemic (two words)
8   A therapy used to deliver aerosolized medication periodically with positive pressure breaths (abbreviation)
9   Another name for bilevel continuous positive airway pressure (CPAP) ventilators (abbreviation)
10  A symptom of chronic hypoventilation
14  A type of sleep apnea that originates in the brain
15  A setting that allows positive-pressure levels to gradually increase
17  Medication given to treat gastric insufflation
19  A type of heated humidifier that has been shown to reduce drying of the nasal mucosa during NIV
21  A type of mask that covers both the nose and the mouth
22  Abbreviation for a type of pneumonia acquired outside the hospital
23  The material that fastens the head gear

### Down

1   A type of pulmonary edema due to a weak heart
3   Uses a pressure-targeted ventilator and a mask (abbreviation)
4   Noninvasive positive-pressure ventilation (abbreviation)
5   A type of hypoventilation that occurs at night
6   Type of sleep apnea that occurs from the collapse of the upper airway during sleep
7   A portable negative-pressure device (two words)
11  The setting that controls the amount of time it takes for the positive-pressure level to gradually increase (two words)
12  The expiratory setting for bilevel CPAP (abbreviation)
13  Right-sided heart failure due to an obstructive pulmonary disease (two words)
16  Secretions that are dried up are
18  The inspiratory setting for bilevel CPAP (abbreviation)

**CHAPTER REVIEW QUESTIONS**

1. Define *NIV.*
   _____
   _____

2. What are the three basic methods of applying NIV?
   a. _____
   b. _____
   c. _____

3. Explain how negative-pressure ventilators work.
   _____
   _____
   _____
   _____
   _____

4. Name two negative-pressure ventilators.
   a. _____
   b. _____

5. What is the most significant benefit of NIV?
   _____

6. What is the primary goal of NIV in the acute care setting?
   _____

7. List six clinical benefits of NIV in the acute care setting.
   a. _____
   b. _____
   c. _____
   d. _____
   e. _____

8. List three clinical benefits of NIV in the chronic care setting.
   a. _____
   b. _____
   c. _____

9. Describe how the use of NIV in acute respiratory failure improves gas exchange.
   _____
   _____

10. Explain the benefits of using NIV via a facemask instead of invasive mechanical ventilation in the treatment of acute respiratory failure due to chronic obstructive pulmonary disease (COPD).
    _____
    _____
    _____

11. What benefit was seen when using NIV for COPD patients with community-acquired pneumonia (CAP)?
    _____
    _____

12. When a patient with cardiogenic pulmonary edema does not respond to conventional pharmacologic and oxygen therapy, what types of NIV have been shown to be effective?
    _____
    _____
    _____

13. List four clinical disorders that manifest in chronic respiratory failure and require NIV as supportive therapy.
    a. _____
    b. _____
    c. _____
    d. _____

14. List five symptoms of chronic hypoventilation.
    a. _____
    b. _____
    c. _____
    d. _____
    e. _____

15. Approximately how many hours must a patient with chronic hypoventilation use NIV to achieve clinical benefits?
    _____

16. Describe the clinical benefits of using NIV only at night or intermittently during the day for patients with neuromuscular disorders.
    _____
    _____
    _____
    _____

17. List the criteria for using NIV with patients who have chronic stable COPD.

_____

_____

_____

18. Lily is a 22-year-old patient with advanced cystic fibrosis. She asks you if NIV could benefit her. How would you respond?

_____

_____

19. What may be the next course of treatment for an OSA patient that continues to hypoventilate and experience nocturnal desaturation while receiving CPAP?

_____

_____

20. Mrs. T is concerned you are attempting to remove her husband from invasive ventilation too soon. She is worried he may become short of breath again, despite the physician's assurance he is ready. How could you explain to her the benefits of reducing the number of days her husband is invasively ventilated?

_____

_____

_____

21. What role does NIV play in "end-of-life" situations?

_____

_____

_____

22. List five indications for the use of NIV for adult patients with acute respiratory failure.
    a. _____
    b. _____
    c. _____
    d. _____
    e. _____

23. List the signs and symptoms of respiratory distress in patients who may require ventilatory assistance. Include the arterial blood gas criteria as well.

_____

_____

24. You are the respiratory therapist (RT) working in the emergency department (ED) of a level 1 trauma center when a 28-year-old patient is brought in via emergency medical services with a possible head injury. He is confused, tachypneic, tachycardic, and hemodynamically unstable. Would you suggest NIV to the trauma surgeon? Why or why not?

_____

_____

_____

_____

25. What is the final consideration in the selection of patients with acute respiratory failure for NIV?

_____

26. What are the physiologic criteria for the institution of NIV for patients with severe stable COPD in a chronic care setting?

_____

_____

27. How do portable pressure-targeted ventilators maintain pressure levels and flush exhaled gases from the circuit?

_____

28. What are the trigger, limit, and cycle variables for bilevel PAP (BiPAP)?

_____

_____

29. What are the inspiratory and expiratory settings on the BiPAP called?

_____

30. The typical ranges for the inspiratory and expiratory settings on the BiPAP are

_____.

31. Most pressure-targeted ventilators offer what modes of ventilatory support?

_____

32. What determines the patient's tidal volume during the use of a pressure-targeted ventilator?

_____

_____

33. Where is the source for unintentional leaks in a pressure-targeted ventilator?

_____

34. What makes the pressure-targeted ventilators able to flow trigger, even though there are intentional and unintentional leaks in the system?

35. Explain how average volume assured pressure support (AVAPS) devices work.

36. What patient population may AVAPS be useful?

37. List four factors that cause the $F_IO_2$ for a portable pressure-targeted ventilator to be variable.
   a.
   b.
   c.
   d.

38. How can precise oxygen concentrations be delivered through a pressure-targeted ventilator (PTV)?

39. How can $CO_2$ rebreathing be minimized with a PTV?

40. List the advantages and disadvantages of using an adult acute care ventilator for NIV.

41. When using an adult acute care ventilator for NIV, which mode will make the patient most comfortable and why?

42. Why is it important for heated humidity to be added during NIV?

43. What type of heated humidifier is recommended for NIV? Why?

44. What advantages does the nasal mask have over the full face mask during the administration of NIV?

45. List two common disadvantages of the nasal mask.
   a.
   b.

46. What are the major concerns about using the full face mask and total face mask for the administration of NIV?

47. How much dead space volume does a full face mask have?

48. In what position should the patient be when NIV is being initiated?

49. After ensuring proper mask size and fit, what steps should be taken to initiate NIV?

50. What clinical indicators demonstrate improvement in patient comfort?

51. What measures can be taken to ensure patient comfort when the clinical indicators are absent?

52. What tidal volume range should be used with NIV? How is volume manipulated?

_____

_____

_____

_____

53. When should attempts at the use of NIV be terminated in favor of more invasive measures?

_____

_____

_____

54. What factors affect aerosol delivery during NIV?

_____

_____

_____

55. What problems do nasal masks or full face masks present during aerosol delivery?

_____

_____

56. What causes pressure sores on the nasal bridge, and what can be done to alleviate this problem?

_____

_____

_____

_____

57. What can be done to reduce gastric insufflation during NIV?

_____

_____

_____

58. List the five most serious complications of NIV.

a. _____

b. _____

c. _____

d. _____

e. _____

59. What are the common methods of weaning a patient from NIV?

_____

## CRITICAL THINKING QUESTIONS

1. Describe a clinical situation that would cause an NIV *not* to trigger from expiratory positive airway pressure (EPAP) to inspiratory positive airway pressure breathing (IPAP) or cycle from IPAP to EPAP?

_____

_____

_____

2. What are the issues that lead to patient noncompliance with NIV, and how can they be alleviated?

_____

_____

_____

3. Describe how placement of the leak port and oxygen bleed-in affects the $F_IO_2$ delivered to the patient through NIV.

_____

_____

_____

_____

_____

_____

_____

## CASE STUDIES

### Case Study 1

A 68-year-old male is currently in the ED being seen for what appears to be an exacerbation of congestive heart failure. He is oriented to person, place, and time, but is very anxious. Physical examination findings are as follows: pulse 129 beats/min and thready; blood pressure 108/64 mm Hg; temperature 37° C; respirations 28 breaths/min, shallow, and labored, with accessory muscle use. Auscultation reveals bilateral decreased breath sounds with diffuse coarse crackles on inspiration. The patient has no cough and is diaphoretic. The respiratory therapist places the patient on a non-rebreather mask and draws an arterial blood gas (ABG) after 15 minutes. The ABG shows pH 7.31, $PaCO_2$ 49 mm Hg, $P_aO_2$ 53 mm Hg, $S_aO_2$ 86%, and $HCO_3^-$ 23 mEq/L.

1. Does this patient meet the selection criteria for NIV? Why or why not?

_____

_____

_____

2. If NIV is appropriate, what settings should be used? If not, what other respiratory therapy should be initiated?

_____

_____

_____

After 3 hours of treatment, the patient has become agitated, confused, and uncooperative.

3. What action should be taken at this time?

_____

_____

_____

## Case Study 2

A 75-year-old man with a long history of COPD and a past smoking history of 114 pack-years presents to the ED with shortness of breath, productive cough with green purulent sputum, and cyanosis. He has had two prior hospitalizations for acute infective exacerbations of his COPD within the past year. He has no comorbidities or occupational exposure. Physical examination reveals the following: pulse 105 beats/min and regular, blood pressure 140/85 mm Hg, and respirations 30 breaths/min with prolonged expiration and use of accessory muscles; percussion is hyper-resonant, breath sounds are reduced bilaterally with prolonged expiratory wheezes. Laboratory work shows white blood cells (WBCs) 11,500 cells/$mm_3$ and room air ABG pH 7.30, $PaCO_2$ 55 mm Hg, $P_aO_2$ 53 mm Hg, and $HCO_3^-$ 32 mEq/L.

1. Analyze this situation and identify and explain five presenting problems.

_____

_____

_____

_____

_____

2. What treatment recommendations should be suggested for this patient at this time?

_____

_____

_____

_____

_____

A repeat ABG following appropriate therapy reveals the following: pH 7.19, PaCO$_2$ 67 mm Hg, and P$_a$O$_2$ 60 mm Hg.

3. What is the most appropriate treatment option at this time?

_____

_____

_____

## NBRC-STYLE QUESTIONS

1. Symptoms of chronic hypoventilation include which of the following?
   1. Fatigue
   2. Morning headache
   3. Hypoxemia
   4. Insomnia
   a. 1 and 2 only
   b. 2 and 3 only
   c. 3 and 4 only
   d. 1 and 4 only

2. A male COPD patient, 5 feet 10 inches tall, has been placed on NIV with an IPAP of 8 cm H$_2$O and an EPAP of 4 cm H$_2$O. The patient's exhaled volume was measured at 350 mL, and the ABGs on this setting were pH 7.27, PaCO$_2$ 77 mm Hg, P$_a$O$_2$ 50 mm Hg, and base excess +7. The most appropriate action is which of the following?
   a. Increase the EPAP to 6 cm H$_2$O.
   b. Increase the IPAP to 10 cm H$_2$O.
   c. Decrease the IPAP to 6 cm H$_2$O.
   d. Bleed in 4 L/min of oxygen.

3. The target tidal volume for a patient with an ideal body weight of 58 kg, who is receiving NIV, is which of the following?
   a. 250 mL
   b. 350 mL
   c. 500 mL
   d. 700 mL

4. The respiratory therapist notices that there has been a drop in the exhaled tidal volume of a patient receiving NIV. The most appropriate action to take is which of the following?
   a. Increase the IPAP
   b. Decrease the EPAP
   c. Adjust the interface
   d. Change the tubing

5. A patient with chronic hypercapnic respiratory failure is currently using NIV only at night, with the following parameters: assist mode IPAP 9 cm H$_2$O and EPAP 4 cm H$_2$O. The patient is noted to be short of breath with a spontaneous rate of 25 breaths/min. The action that will alleviate this problem is which of the following?
   a. Switch to the control mode.
   b. Increase the IPAP percentage to 35%.
   c. Decrease the EPAP to 2 cm H$_2$O.
   d. Increase the IPAP to 11 cm H$_2$O.

6. Which of the following situations will provide the highest oxygen concentration to a patient who is using a portable pressure-targeted ventilator?
   a. Low IPAP and EPAP settings
   b. High IPAP and EPAP settings
   c. Leak port and oxygen bleed-in at the mask
   d. Leak port and oxygen bleed-in in the circuit

7. The most appropriate type of humidifier to use with NIV is which of the following?
   a. Wick-type humidifier
   b. Heat moisture exchanger
   c. Heated bubble humidifier
   d. Heated passover-type humidifier

8. Which of the following will reduce a significant air leak through the mouth of a patient who is receiving NIV via a nose mask?
   a. Using a chin strap
   b. Adding a forehead spacer
   c. Switching to nasal pillows
   d. Tightening the headgear straps

9. A patient is receiving mask CPAP with 8 cm H$_2$O and 80% oxygen. The ABG on this setting is pH 7.37, PaCO$_2$ 37 mm Hg, and P$_a$O$_2$ 55 mm Hg. The most appropriate recommendation is which of the following?
   a. Increase the F$_I$O$_2$ to 90%.
   b. Intubate and mechanically ventilate.
   c. Increase the CPAP level to 12 cm H$_2$O.
   d. Switch to bilevel positive-pressure ventilation.

10. A patient with which of the following problems should be excluded from a trial with NIV?
    a. Amyotrophic lateral sclerosis
    b. Cardiogenic pulmonary edema
    c. Hemodynamically unstable acute respiratory distress syndrome
    d. CAP

# 20 Weaning and Discontinuation From Mechanical Ventilation

## LEARNING OBJECTIVES

*Upon completion of this chapter, the reader will be able to do the following:*

1. List the weaning parameters and acceptable values for ventilator discontinuation.
2. Compare the three standard modes of weaning in relation to their success in discontinuing ventilation.
3. Define the closed-loop modes of weaning described in the chapter.
4. Recognize appropriate use of closed-loop modes of weaning based on the description of a clinical setting.
5. Identify assessment criteria for discontinuing a spontaneous breathing trial in a clinical situation.
6. Describe criteria used to determine whether a patient is ready for extubation.
7. Recognize postextubation difficulties from a clinical case description.
8. Recommend appropriate treatment for postextubation difficulties.
9. State the first recommendation for weaning a patient from mechanical ventilation established by the task force formed by the American College of Chest Physicians, the Society of Critical Care Medicine, and the American Association for Respiratory Care.
10. Describe an appropriate treatment for a patient with an irreversible respiratory disorder that requires long-term ventilation.
11. Name the parameter used as the primary index of drive to breathe.
12. Suggest adjustments to ventilator settings during use of a standard weaning mode based on patient assessment.
13. Explain the appropriate procedure for management of a patient for whom a spontaneous breathing trial has failed.
14. Explain the function of long-term care facilities in the management of ventilator-dependent patients.
15. Assess data used to establish the probable cause of failure to wean.

**KEY TERMS CROSSWORD PUZZLE**

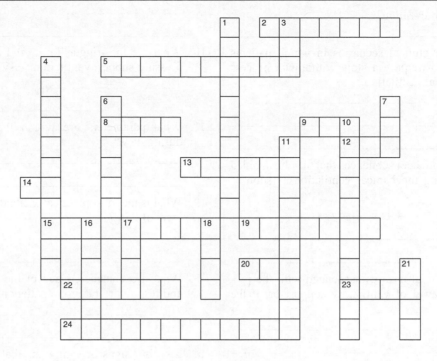

## Across

2 Type of epinephrine used to treat airway edema following extubation
5 Area of edema that may occur after the endotracheal tube (ET) is removed
8 The gradual reduction in support
9 A non-physician-directed protocol (abbreviation)
12 A mode designed to make automatic adjustments from the time ventilation is initiated until ventilation can be discontinued (abbreviation)
13 Adapter used during a T-piece weaning from mechanical ventilation
14 Volume-targeted pressure support (abbreviation)
15 Respiratory _____ is the altering use of the diaphragm and accessory muscles in order to breath
19 A postextubation sound heard when subglottic edema is present
20 Trial of sustained breathing without mechanical support (abbreviation)
22 A low-density gas mixture
23 Index that evaluates compliance, respiratory rate, oxygenation, and inspiratory pressure (abbreviation)
24 Placement of an ET tube following the recent removal of it

## Down

1 Removal of the ET tube
3 A feature intensive care unit (ICU) ventilators have to deliver exactly the amount of pressure required to overcome the resistive load imposed by the ET (abbreviation)
4 A type of spasm that may occur after the ET tube is removed
6 This psychological factor is high when patients are optimistic and motivated to recover.
7 This can be added to spontaneous breaths to reduce the work of breathing (WOB) (abbreviation).
10 Type of breathing in which the chest wall moves in during inspiration and out during exhalation
11 Associated with a suppressed gag or cough reflex
16 A type of breathing trial
17 Index for ventilatory muscle capability that is calculated using the frequency and tidal volume (abbreviation)
18 This psychological factor is high when patients lie passively in bed.
21 Ventilation without an ET (abbreviation)

**CHAPTER REVIEW QUESTIONS**

1. Define the term *weaning*.

   _____

2. Describe three clinical scenarios in which patients typically do not require a slow withdrawal process from mechanical ventilation.

   a. _____

   b. _____

   c. _____

3. List three potential consequences that may be avoided by discontinuing mechanical ventilation as soon as possible.

   a. _____

   b. _____

   c. _____

4. List three potential hazards associated with the premature withdrawal of ventilatory support or of the airway.

   a. _____

   b. _____

   c. _____

5. List three approaches commonly used to reduce ventilatory support.

   a. _____

   b. _____

   c. _____

6. Closed-loop modes used for weaning patients include the following:

   _____

   _____

7. What should be the primary factor in determining whether a patient is ready to be weaned from mechanical ventilation?

   _____

8. Describe the underlying theory of intermittent mandatory ventilation (IMV) that helps facilitate the weaning of a patient from mechanical ventilation.

   _____

   _____

9. Why is pressure support (PS) added during IMV?

   _____

   _____

10. What are the trigger, limit, and cycle variables for pressure-support ventilation (PSV)?

    _____

    _____

11. What parameters are within the patient's control during PSV?

    _____

    _____

12. What is the most practical method of establishing the level of PSV?

    _____

    _____

13. What are considered acceptable ranges for the $V_T$ and respiratory rate for a patient receiving PSV?

    _____

    _____

14. List four signs or symptoms that would indicate an inappropriately set PS level.

    _____

    _____

    _____

15. What is the major disadvantage of T-piece weaning?

    _____

    _____

16. (a) What mode of mechanical ventilation can be used as a substitute for T-piece weaning?

    _____

    (b) What is the major advantage of using this mode instead of a T-piece trial?

    _____

17. In the following list, match the description with the appropriate weaning mode.

| Weaning Mode | Description |
|---|---|
| _____ ATC | (a) Allows spontaneous breathing between mechanical breaths |
| _____ VS | (b) Similar to a T-piece with alarm support capability |
| _____ MMV | (c) Compensates for increased resistance and WOB through an ET |
| _____ ASV | (d) Adjusts to various levels of support automatically |
| _____ Automode | (e) Allows patient control of the rate, time, and depth of each breath |
| _____ IMV | (f) Provides pressure-limited breaths that target a volume and rate |
| _____ PSV | (g) Maintains a consistent minimum minute ventilation |
| _____ CPAP | (h) Delivers a set VT in a pressure mode of ventilation |

18. List three clinical criteria for weaning.
    a. _____
    b. _____
    c. _____

19. List four psychological factors that may adversely affect the weaning process.
    a. _____
    b. _____
    c. _____
    d. _____

20. Your patient's total parenteral nutrition was set inappropriately low while receiving mechanical ventilation. What implications does this have for her ability to be weaned from mechanical ventilation?
    _____
    _____
    _____

21. Describe the procedure for a cuff leak test.
    _____
    _____

22. In a cuff leak test, what does the measured volume that escapes from around a deflated cuff indicate?
    _____
    _____

23. Why is vital capacity not considered a good indicator for discontinuation of ventilator support?
    _____
    _____

24. What parameter is a primary index of the inspiratory drive to breathe?
    _____

25. A _____ (high; low) oxygen cost of breathing and a(an) _____ (increased; decreased) metabolic rate may result in increased WOB.

26. (a) What index is used to assess the potential for respiratory muscle overload and fatigue?
    _____

    (b) What four components does this index measure?
    1. _____
    2. _____
    3. _____
    4. _____

27. (a) Calculate the index that evaluates compliance, respiratory rate, oxygenation, and inspiratory pressure (CROP index) using these data: $C_D = 20$ mL/cm $H_2O$, $P_{Imax} = 25$ cm $H_2O$, $P_aO_2 = 70$ mm Hg, $P_AO_2 = 100$ mm Hg, rate = 18 breaths/min.
    _____
    _____
    _____

    (b) Does this value indicate the possibility of successful ventilator withdrawal? Give your reasons.
    _____

28. How long must a patient tolerate a spontaneous breathing trial (SBT) to be considered ready for ventilator discontinuation and extubation?
    _____

29. What is the formula for the rapid shallow breathing index (RSBI)?
    _____

30. Calculate the RSBI, given the following values: $V_T = 600\,mL$, rate = 26 breaths/min.
_____

31. What values of a RSBI indicate that weaning may be successful?
_____

32. List the two criteria that must be met before a decision can be made to remove an artificial airway.
    a. _____
    b. _____

33. List four factors that indicate extubation is likely to be successful.
    a. _____
    b. _____
    c. _____
    d. _____

34. List three clinical patient conditions in which an artificial airway should not be removed after weaning from mechanical ventilation.
    a. _____
    b. _____
    c. _____

35. List three complications associated with prolonged intubation.
    a. _____
    b. _____
    c. _____

36. How does administration of heliox aid the treatment of partial airway obstruction and stridor caused by postextubation glottic edema?
    a. _____
    b. _____
    c. _____

37. How is heliox therapy administered in this situation?
_____

38. List six factors that can increase the risk of aspiration after extubation.
    a. _____
    b. _____
    c. _____
    d. _____
    e. _____
    f. _____

39. What is the primary indication for noninvasive positive-pressure ventilation (NIV) after extubation?
_____
_____

40. List five benefits of using NIV after extubation.
    a. _____
    b. _____
    c. _____
    d. _____
    e. _____

41. List the criteria for instituting NIV when an extubated patient is unable to sustain adequate ventilation.
_____
_____
_____
_____
_____

42. List four types of medication that can depress the central ventilatory drive.
    a. _____
    b. _____
    c. _____
    d. _____

43. Explain the advantages of therapist-driven protocols for both patients and hospital staff.
_____
_____
_____

44. List the clinical characteristics of patients that may benefit from a tracheostomy tube placement.
_____
_____
_____
_____
_____

45. List five beneficial outcomes for performing a tracheotomy.
    a. _____
    b. _____
    c. _____
    d. _____
    e. _____

46. What alternative sites are available for patients who are medically stable, yet still require mechanical ventilation following multiple failed weaning attempts in the ICU?

_____

_____

_____

_____

47. List five goals for weaning in long-term care facilities.

a. _____

b. _____

c. _____

d. _____

e. _____

## CRITICAL THINKING QUESTIONS

For Questions 1 and 2, refer to the following scenario.

A patient is successfully weaned from mechanical ventilatory support. A leak test is performed before extubation, and the measured volume is 80 mL.

1. What can the respiratory therapist conclude from this finding?

_____

_____

_____

2. What should the respiratory therapist recommend before extubation?

_____

_____

3. Ten minutes after a patient was extubated, the respiratory therapist hears marked stridor, increased WOB, intercostal retractions, and a 20% drop in the $SpO_2$. An aerosolized racemic epinephrine treatment is given, but no effect is noted. What should the therapist recommend?

_____

_____

_____

4. You are discussing the best mode of weaning a patient from mechanical ventilation with the attending physician, who prefers to use IMV as a means of weaning patients. You would like to try PSV on this patient. The physician asks you why? Explain why you would choose PSV by comparing and contrasting it to IMV.

_____

_____

## CASE STUDIES

### Case Study 1

While monitoring a patient 10 minutes after initiation of a T-piece trial through the ventilator, the respiratory therapist observes increased restlessness, an increase in the respiratory rate from 16 to 36 breaths/min, with paradoxical chest movement and use of accessory muscles, and an increase in the heart rate from 80 to 120 beats/min.

1. What may be the primary reason for this patient's failed weaning attempt?

_____

_____

_____

2. What would be the most appropriate action to take at this time?

_____

_____

_____

## Case Study 2

A 45-year-old male trauma patient has been maintained on volume-controlled ventilation for approximately 2 weeks. The patient's overall condition is improving, but he is not totally alert, and he has periods of apnea. The physician would like to start weaning the patient from the ventilator.

1. What weaning modalities should the therapist recommend and why?

   _____

   _____

   _____

   _____

## Case Study 3

A 65-year-old patient, who suffered a myocardial infarction several days ago, is being ventilated in a volume control mode at a set rate of 12 breaths/min and a $V_T$ of 600 mL. The patient's condition is currently stable, and his overall condition is improving. The physician asks the respiratory therapist to initiate a weaning trial; the results are as follows.

| Mode | IMV |
|------|-----|
| Mandatory rate | 6 breaths/min |
| Mandatory $V_T$ | 600 mL |
| Spontaneous rate | 35 breaths/min |
| Spontaneous $V_T$ | 185 mL |

1. What is the cause of the high spontaneous respiratory rate?

   _____

   _____

   _____

   _____

2. What are the therapist's options at this point?

   _____

   _____

   _____

## NBRC-STYLE QUESTIONS

1. In the assessment of a patient's respiratory rate, which of the following values would indicate the highest probability that the patient will likely be able to maintain spontaneous ventilation?
   a. Less than 45 breaths/min
   b. Less than 40 breaths/min
   c. Less than 30 breaths/min
   d. Less than 25 breaths/min

2. Which of the following drugs is used most often to treat postextubation glottic edema?
   a. Racemic epinephrine
   b. Intravenous steroids
   c. Albuterol via metered-dose inhaler
   d. Cromolyn sodium

3. Which of the following is the minimal acceptable range for maximal inspiratory pressure when assessing ventilatory muscle strength?
   a. $-5$ to $-10$ cm $H_2O$
   b. $-10$ to $-15$ cm $H_2O$
   c. $-20$ to $-30$ cm $H_2O$
   d. $-40$ to $-50$ cm $H_2O$
4. A patient is being weaned from mechanical ventilation. The ventilator settings and arterial blood gas results are as follows.

   | Mode | IMV |
   | --- | --- |
   | Set rate | 8 breaths/min |
   | $V_T$ | 650 mL |
   | $F_IO_2$ | 0.35 |
   | PS | 25 cm $H_2O$ |
   | PH | 7.44 |
   | PaCO$_2$ | 34 mm Hg |
   | P$_a$O$_2$ | 96 mm Hg |

   Based on this information, what should the respiratory therapist recommend?
   a. Increase the synchronized IMV rate
   b. Reduce the PS level
   c. Reduce the $V_T$
   d. Reduce the $F_IO_2$
5. Which of the following statements is true?
   a. In IMV, all breaths are spontaneously triggered.
   b. In the A/C mode, every patient effort delivers the set $V_T$.
   c. In IMV, all breaths deliver the same $V_T$.
   d. PS can be used to augment the $V_T$ in A/C.
6. A patient is being weaned in the MMV mode. The MMV is set at 7 L and the patient is breathing at a rate of 14 breaths/min with a spontaneous $V_T$ of 600 mL. How much ventilatory assistance is the ventilator providing?
   a. Minute ventilation of 4 L
   b. No assistance required
   c. Respiratory rate of 8 breaths/min
   d. Minute ventilation of 7 L

7. Which of the following would indicate a successful weaning trial and extubation?
   1. P$_a$O$_2$ 80 mm Hg on $F_IO_2 \leq 0.4$
   2. P$_a$O$_2$/$F_IO_2$ ratio $\leq 150$ to 200 mm Hg
   3. Dopamine greater than 5 mg/kg/min to maintain blood pressure
   4. pH 7.38
   a. 1
   b. 2, 3, and 4
   c. 1 and 4
   d. 2, 3, and 4
8. Which of the following modes of mechanical ventilation automatically adjusts ventilatory parameters based on continuous monitoring of compliance and airway resistance?
   1. Proportional assist ventilation
   2. Pressure-regulated volume control
   3. Adaptive support ventilation
   4. Airway pressure release ventilation
   a. 1 and 2
   b. 1 and 3
   c. 1, 2, and 4
   d. 2, 3, and 4
9. Which of the following should be required before an SBT?
   1. The patient should be given a sedative.
   2. The patient should be able to maintain an adequate P$_a$O$_2$ and P$_a$CO$_2$ during spontaneous breathing.
   3. The patient should be hemodynamically stable.
   4. The patient's P$_{Imax}$ should be 50 mm Hg.
   a. 1 and 4
   b. 1, 2, and 3
   c. 2, 3, and 4
   d. 2 and 3
10. Which of the following parameters indicates that an SBT will likely be successful?
    a. Minute ventilation of 14 L
    b. P$_a$O$_2$ of 55 mm Hg on an $F_IO_2$ of 0.5
    c. V$_D$/V$_T$ ratio of 0.7
    d. P$_a$O$_2$/$F_IO_2$ ratio of 280 mm Hg

# 21 Long-Term Ventilation

## LEARNING OBJECTIVES

*Upon completion of this chapter, the reader will be able to do the following:*

1. State the goals of mechanical ventilation in a home environment.
2. List the criteria for selection of patients suitable for successful homecare ventilation.
3. Name the factors used to estimate the cost of home mechanical ventilation.
4. Describe facilities used for the care of patients requiring extended ventilator management in terms of type of care provided and cost.
5. Identify the factors used when considering selection of a ventilator for home use.
6. Compare the criteria for discharging a child versus discharging an adult who is ventilator dependent.
7. Explain the use of the following noninvasive ventilation techniques: pneumobelt, chest cuirass, full-body chamber (tank ventilator), and body suit (jacket ventilator).
8. List follow-up assessment techniques used with patients on home ventilation.
9. Describe some of the difficulties families experience when caring for a patient in the home.
10. Identify pieces of equipment that are essential to accomplishing intermittent positive pressure ventilation in the home.
11. Name the specific equipment needed for patients in the home who cannot be without ventilator support.
12. Name the appropriate modes used with first-generation portable/homecare ventilators.
13. On the basis of a patient's assessment and ventilator parameters, name the operational features required for that patient's home ventilator and any additional equipment that will be needed.
14. Discuss the instructions given to the patient and caregivers when preparing a patient for discharge home.
15. List the items that should appear in a monthly report of patients on home mechanical ventilation.
16. Describe patients who would benefit from continuous positive airway pressure by nasal mask or pillows.
17. Recommend solutions to potential complications and side effects of nasal mask continuous positive airway pressure.
18. Recognize from a clinical example a potential complication of negative pressure ventilation.
19. Name three methods of improving secretion clearance besides suctioning.
20. List the advantages of using mechanical insufflation-exsufflation in conjunction with positive pressure ventilation.
21. List five psychological problems that can occur in ventilator-assisted individuals.
22. Explain the procedure for accomplishing speech in ventilator-assisted individuals.
23. Compare the functions of the Portex and the Pittsburg speaking tracheostomy tubes.
24. Name one essential step required by the respiratory therapist when setting up a speaking valve for a ventilator-assisted individual.
25. List six circumstances in which speaking devices may be contraindicated.

**KEY TERMS CROSSWORD PUZZLE**

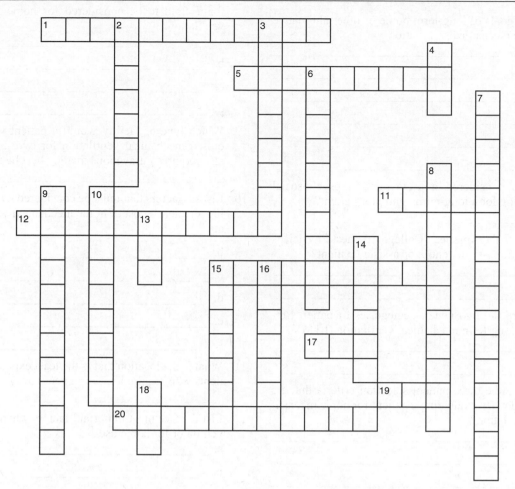

**Across**

1 Easy to understand and manipulate (two words)
5 Reflux can cause this to erode
11 An obstruction of the intestinal tract associated with immobility of the bowel or a mechanical blockage
12 To remove a tracheostomy tube
15 These must vibrate to produce a voice (two words)
17 Homecare equipment supplier (abbreviation)
19 Mechanical cough machine (abbreviation)
20 Type of tube that goes into the stomach

**Down**

2 Temporary relief for the caregiver
3 Type of planning team
4 Type of sleep disorder (abbreviation)
6 Intermittent abdominal pressure ventilator
7 Type of breathing used to assist patients with poor respiratory muscle strength, also called "frog" breathing
8 Type of tracheostomy tube with an extra opening
9 Surgical opening between the jejunum and the surface of the abdominal wall
10 Type of speaking valve (two words)
13 Opposite of PPV (abbreviation)
14 A speaking tracheostomy tube that has an opening in the posterior portion above the cuff
15 Homecare disinfectant
16 Type of ventilation indicated in 13 down
18 Ventilator-assisted individuals (abbreviation)

## CHAPTER REVIEW QUESTIONS

1. List six goals of long-term home or other alternative care site mechanical ventilation.
   a. _____
   b. _____
   c. _____
   d. _____
   e. _____
   f. _____

2. What is considered improvement in psychosocial well-being for a long-term ventilator patient?
   _____

3. How does the American College of Chest Physicians define a long-term ventilator-assisted patient?
   _____
   _____

4. What are the two general categories of patients requiring long-term mechanical ventilation (LTMV)?
   a. _____
   b. _____

5. What are the three patient selection criteria that are assessed when evaluating a patient for home mechanical ventilation?
   a. _____
   b. _____
   c. _____

6. What types of patients are most likely to be successful with long-term ventilation?
   _____
   _____
   _____
   _____

7. Describe the clinical factors you would assess prior to recommending a patient for LTMV in the home or in a long-term care facility.
   _____
   _____

8. List four additional criteria must be considered for a child to be considered for home mechanical ventilation.
   a. _____
   b. _____
   c. _____
   d. _____

9. Which type of facility would a patient who has required mechanical ventilation for over 30 days and also requires intravenous therapy best be treated?
   _____

10. List six factors that must be considered when estimating a patient's cost of home mechanical ventilation.
    a. _____
    b. _____
    c. _____
    d. _____
    e. _____
    f. _____

11. What is the location that is the least expensive for patients who require long-term ventilatory care?
    _____

12. List the five most important factors when choosing a ventilator for home use.
    a. _____
    b. _____
    c. _____
    d. _____
    e. _____

13. What backup equipment is necessary for a patient requiring LTMV at home? What is the rationale for each?

    **Backup Equipment**          **Rationale**

    _____          _____
    _____          _____
    _____          _____

14. What is the rationale for the increased level of follow-up and evaluation of the ventilatory status of children maintained on mechanical ventilation at home as compared with adults?

    _____

    _____

15. Identify three classifications of ventilator-dependent patients.

    a. _____

    b. _____

    c. _____

16. List four psychosocial factors that must be addressed to ensure a successful transition home for the ventilator-dependent patient.

    a. _____

    b. _____

    c. _____

    d. _____

17. List five factors that must be addressed when evaluating the home environment before discharge of patients requiring mechanical ventilation.

    a. _____

    b. _____

    c. _____

    d. _____

    e. _____

18. Before a patient is discharged to the home care setting, the primary caregiver asks you what difficulties may be experienced when caring for a patient in the home. How would you respond?

    _____

    _____

    _____

19. In addition to the mechanical ventilator and its related equipment, list six of the other equipment/supplies that are needed to support the patient receiving mechanical ventilation in the home.

    a. _____

    b. _____

    c. _____

    d. _____

    e. _____

    f. _____

20. Before discharge, what are the primary skills the respiratory therapist must teach the patient, his or her family, and others involved in the care of the patient?

    _____

    _____

    _____

21. What components must be included in a written monthly report when performing a home visit?

    _____

    _____

    _____

22. List the three electrical power sources used by home ventilators.

    a. _____

    b. _____

    c. _____

23. List three contraindications for the use of negative-pressure ventilators.

    a. _____

    b. _____

    c. _____

24. Explain why a patient receiving mechanical ventilation with oxygen and positive end-expiratory pressure (PEEP) in the home may encounter difficulty triggering the ventilator.

    _____

    _____

    _____

25. What are some of the advantages of providing home mechanical ventilation with the newer (second-generation) portable home care ventilators?

_____

_____

_____

_____

26. List the four most common gastrointestinal disorders associated with patients receiving LTMV.

a. _____

b. _____

c. _____

d. _____

27. A substantial number of patients who transfer to long-term care facilities on mechanical ventilation have what type of disorder?

_____

28. List three factors that contribute to psychological problems in VAIs.

a. _____

b. _____

c. _____

29. How do the rocking bed and pneumobelt support spontaneous ventilation?

_____

_____

30. What patient conditions are contraindications for use of the rocking bed?

_____

_____

31. What type of patient would benefit from a rocking bed as a form of ventilatory support?

_____

32. In what type of therapy is the phrenic nerve stimulated through surgically implanted electrodes?

_____

33. What happens to a patient with obstructive sleep apnea (OSA) during sleep?

_____

_____

34. List three goals of CPAP therapy when used to treat OSA.

a. _____

b. _____

c. _____

35. What patient interfaces are available for delivering CPAP therapy?

_____

_____

36. What are the complications associated with CPAP therapy?

_____

_____

_____

37. What are the physical requirements a patient needs to perform glossopharyngeal breathing?

_____

_____

38. What type of patients benefit from the use of glossopharyngeal breathing?

_____

39. What are the minimum vital capacity and peak cough expiratory flow rate necessary to produce an effective cough?

_____

40. List three techniques that aid in the management of secretions for patients with neuromuscular disease.

a. _____

b. _____

c. _____

41. How is assisted coughing performed?

_____

_____

42. What are the advantages of mechanical insufflation-exsufflation (MI-E) compared with tracheal suctioning?

43. In what type of patients is MI-E contraindicated?

44. What type of tracheostomy tube should a therapist recommend for a patient who is unable to speak and at risk of aspiration?

45. What type of tracheostomy tube should a therapist recommend for a patient who has no trouble swallowing and can breathe for long periods of time?

46. In addition to deflating the cuff, what ventilator parameters can be adjusted to help a patient produce speech or to improve the speech quality?

47. What are the potential hazards of cuff deflation of VAIs?

48. Before a cuff is deflated to allow for speaking, what should the patient be evaluated for?

49. What devices are available to allow VAIs to speak?

50. How does a Passy-Muir speaking valve allow for speech in the patient with a tracheostomy, who is receiving mechanical ventilation?

51. List three clinical circumstances in which the use of speaking devices may be contraindicated.
    a.
    b.
    c.

52. Compare the functions of the Portex and the Pitt speaking tracheostomy tubes.

53. What steps need to be taken prior to setting up a speaking valve for a VAI?

54. What is the most cost-effective disinfecting solution available for home care patients to disinfect their equipment?

55. How long must water be boiled before it can be used in a humidifier?

**CRITICAL THINKING QUESTIONS**

Questions 1 and 2 refer to the following scenario.

After undergoing a sleep study, a patient diagnosed with OSA is prescribed CPAP via nasal mask. During a follow-up visit by the therapist, the patient states that his sleep is not improving and that he is experiencing eye irritation.

1. What could be the cause of the patient's problem?

2. What steps can the therapist take to alleviate the situation?

Question 3 refers to the following scenario.

A VAI in a long-term [A1] care facility is being maintained on pressure support ventilation. The respiratory therapist is asked to evaluate the patient to see if he can tolerate a speaking valve. After cuff deflation, and before attaching the valve, the patient suddenly becomes short of breath, with an increase in the heart rate.

3. What could have brought on the sudden onset of respiratory distress?

_____

_____

_____

_____

Question 4 refers to the following scenario.

Fifteen minutes after initiating PEEP with an external threshold resistor for a patient supported by a home care ventilator, the respiratory therapist observes that the patient's respiratory rate has doubled, her tidal volume has dropped significantly, and the ventilator's low-pressure alarm has been activated.

4. What is the probable cause of this problem?

_____

## CASE STUDIES

### Case Study 1

A patient in the early stages of a neuromuscular disease complains to his physician that he is having difficulty sleeping. In addition, he is experiencing headaches and becomes increasingly tired toward the end of the day.

1. What are the possible causes of this patient's symptoms?

_____

2. What type of therapy should the therapist recommend to help treat this patient?

_____

3. What would be the goals of the recommended therapy?

_____

4. How would you evaluate the effectiveness of the therapy?

_____

### Case Study 2

A 70-year-old woman spent 1 month in the hospital for exacerbation of chronic obstructive pulmonary disease (COPD). After numerous attempts at weaning had failed, the patient received a tracheostomy. After careful evaluation, the patient was discharged home on continuous ventilatory support. A follow-up visit was made 2 weeks after discharge. The therapist found the patient to be febrile, auscultation revealed rhonchi in the right upper and middle lobes, and suctioning produced a moderate amount of yellow sputum. The patient was admitted to the hospital and diagnosed with pneumonia.

1. What would be your assessment of why this patient developed a pulmonary infection so soon after discharge?

_____

_____

2. What recommendations, if any, would you make?

_____

_____

## NBRC-STYLE QUESTIONS

1. If a home-care ventilator does not have an $F_IO_2$ control, what is the most common means by which oxygen can be delivered to the patient?
   a. Using an external blender
   b. Using a microprocessor-controlled proportioning valve
   c. Mixing air and oxygen cylinders to approximate the desired $F_IO_2$
   d. Bleeding oxygen into the system through the inspiratory limb

2. In the home setting, how long should suction catheters be soaked in a disinfectant solution?
   a. A minimum of 2 minutes
   b. A minimum of 5 minutes
   c. A minimum of 10 minutes
   d. A minimum of 25 minutes

3. Which of the following represents the range of CPAP levels available on most home-care units?
   a. 0 to 2.0 cm $H_2O$
   b. 2.5 to 20 cm $H_2O$
   c. 25 to 35 cm $H_2O$
   d. 35 to 45 cm $H_2O$

4. Which of the following patient conditions would exclude them from being treated with negative-pressure ventilation?
   a. Excessive secretions
   b. Neuromuscular disease
   c. Spinal cord injuries
   d. Central hypoventilation syndromes

5. During a follow-up visit of a patient recently started on CPAP therapy by nasal mask, the patient complains of nasal dryness and congestion. Which of the following recommendations would help remedy the problem?
   a. Decrease the flow rate
   b. Decrease the level of CPAP
   c. Add humidification or recommend use of a nasal spray
   d. Readjust the mask to correct for any leaks

6. Which of the following is *not* generally part of a monthly home evaluation?
   a. Vital signs
   b. Pulse oximetry
   c. Bedside pulmonary function studies
   d. Arterial blood gas

7. Contraindications to LTMV include the following:
   a. An $F_IO_2$ requirement greater than 30%
   b. PEEP greater than 5 cm $H_2O$
   c. The need for continuous invasive monitoring
   d. The need for frequent secretion removal

8. Which of the following conditions allow(s) patients certain periods of spontaneous breathing during the day, and generally require(s) only nocturnal ventilatory support?
   1. Myasthenia gravis
   2. End-stage COPD
   3. Kyphoscoliosis
   4. Multiple sclerosis
   a. 1 only
   b. 3 and 4 only
   c. 1, 3, and 4 only
   d. 2, 3, and 4

9. Patient assessment prior to decannulation should include which of the following?
   1. Airway patency
   2. Sufficient muscle strength to generate a cough
   3. Volume and thickness of secretions
   4. Sleep studies
   a. 1 only
   b. 1 and 4 only
   c. 1, 2, and 3 only
   d. 2, 3, and 4

10. Which of the following is not a realistic goal of home mechanical ventilation?
    a. To reverse the disease process
    b. To improve the quality of life
    c. To prolong life
    d. To reduce the number of hospitalizations

# 22 Neonatal and Pediatric Mechanical Ventilation

## LEARNING OBJECTIVES

*Upon completion of this chapter, the reader will be able to do the following:*

1. Discuss the clinical manifestations of respiratory distress in neonatal and pediatric patients.
2. Identify differences in the level of support provided by different forms of noninvasive support.
3. Describe respiratory support device function and settings for different mechanical respiratory support strategies.
4. Identify the primary and secondary goals of ventilatory support of newborn and pediatric patients.
5. Explain some key areas of assessment that influence the decision on whether to initiate ventilatory support.
6. Recognize the indications, goals, limitations, and potentially harmful effects of continuous positive airway pressure (CPAP) in a clinical case.
7. Describe the basic design of nasal devices used to deliver CPAP to an infant.
8. From patient data, recognize the need for mechanical ventilatory support in newborn and pediatric patients.
9. Identify the essential features of a neonatal and pediatric mechanical ventilator.
10. Explain how the advanced features of a ventilator enhance its usefulness over a wide range of clinical settings.
11. Relate the major differences between older-generation neonatal ventilators and modern microprocessor controlled mechanical ventilators.
12. Distinguish demand flow from continuous flow and discuss other modifications that have been made to the basic infant ventilator.
13. Select appropriate ventilator settings based on the patient's weight, diagnosis, and clinical history; also discuss strategies and rationale for ventilator settings.
14. Discuss newborn and pediatric applications, technical aspects, patient management, and cautions for the following ventilatory modes: pressure-controlled ventilation, volume-controlled ventilation, dual-controlled ventilation, pressure support ventilation, airway pressure release ventilation, and neurally adjusted ventilatory assist.
15. Discuss the rationale and indications for high-frequency ventilation (HFV) in newborn and pediatric patients.
16. Compare the characteristics and basic delivery systems of the following HFV techniques: high-frequency positive pressure ventilation, high-frequency jet ventilation, high-frequency flow interruption, high-frequency percussive ventilation, and high-frequency oscillatory ventilation.
17. Explain the physiological and theoretic mechanisms of gas exchange that govern HFV and defend the mechanism thought to be most correct.
18. Explain how settings of a given high-frequency technique are initially adjusted, the effect of individual controls on gas exchange, and strategies of patient management.
19. Discuss the physiological benefits of inhaled nitric oxide therapy and suggest recommended treatment strategies.

**KEY TERMS CROSSWORD PUZZLE**

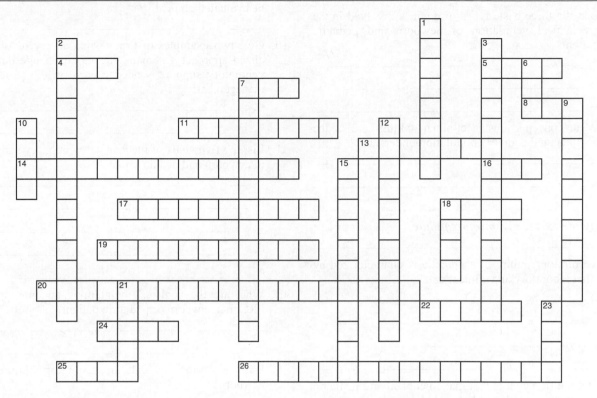

**Across**

4 Condition that is responsive to 24 across (abbreviation)
5 Type of ventilation that uses the highest rates (8 to 20 Hz) (abbreviation)
7 Pulmonary disease of infants; high airway resistance is a major component (abbreviation)
8 Neonatal problem commonly treated with methylxanthines (abbreviation)
11 Type of aspiration syndrome that occurs in term or post-term neonates
13 Abnormal tube-like passage between the trachea and the esophagus
14 A deficiency in the cartilage around a bronchus; leads to atelectasis
16 Infant who weighs 1500 to 2500 g (abbreviation)
17 Type of heart disease present at birth
18 Mode that is unique to infant mechanical ventilation (abbreviation)
19 Congenital split of the roof of the mouth (two words)
20 Incomplete embryologic formation of the diaphragm leads to this (two words)
22 Type of hemoglobin present in a fetus
24 Noninvasive method of increasing functional residual capacity (FRC) and improving lung compliance
25 Mode of ventilation used to percuss the chest to remove secretions (abbreviation)
26 Structure that may remain open after birth (two words)

**Down**

1 Trade name for beractant (a surfactant)
2 Softening of the cartilages of the trachea
3 Failure of the nasopharyngeal (NP) septum to rupture causes this malformation (two words)
6 This sleep disorder is usually treated by 24 across (abbreviation).
7 Viral infection that causes inflammation, swelling, and airway obstruction
9 Exchange of gas between lung units with different time constants
10 Infant weighing less than 1500 g (abbreviation)
12 A selective pulmonary vasodilator used to improve pulmonary blood flow and enhance arterial oxygenation (two words)
15 Interface most often used for application of CPAP (two words)
18 Historically, the mode most often used for infants (abbreviation)
21 Mode that uses frequencies up to 150 breaths/min (abbreviation)
23 An invasive life support procedure (abbreviation)

## CHAPTER REVIEW QUESTIONS

1. List the three basic types of devices involved in the mechanical ventilation of newborn and pediatric patients.
   a. _____
   b. _____
   c. _____

2. What concepts must a clinician taking care of the neonatal and pediatric population understand?
   _____
   _____
   _____

3. Define the term *respiratory failure*.
   _____

4. Respiratory failure in a neonate is characterized by what laboratory and clinical data?
   _____
   _____
   _____
   _____

5. List the five factors that make neonatal and pediatric patients more vulnerable to rapid deterioration.
   a. _____
   b. _____
   c. _____
   d. _____
   e. _____

6. List four signs of respiratory distress in the neonate.
   a. _____
   b. _____
   c. _____
   d. _____
   e. _____

7. Explain *grunting* in a neonatal patient.
   _____
   _____
   _____
   _____

8. How can tissue oxygenation be assessed physically?
   _____
   _____
   _____

9. In what way can oxygen delivery and tissue perfusion be evaluated clinically?
   _____

10. Give two examples of times when a very individualized approach for managing gas exchange during ventilatory support is needed early in the patient's management.
    a. _____
    b. _____

11. List the five goals of mechanical ventilatory support in newborn and pediatric patients.
    a. _____
    b. _____
    c. _____
    d. _____
    e. _____

12. What are the goals of maintaining an appropriate FRC in a newborn or pediatric patient?
    _____
    _____

13. What laboratory data define respiratory failure in newborns?
    _____

14. The minimum acceptable pH for a premature or term newborn is
    _____.

15. What laboratory data define respiratory failure in pediatric patients?
    _____
    _____

16. When maximum oxygen delivery to the tissues is critical, why is fetal hemoglobin not desirable?
    _____
    _____
    _____

17. List the two most common uses for CPAP in pediatric patients.
    a. _____
    b. _____

18. List four clinical situations in which CPAP would be indicated for a neonatal patient.
    a. _____
    b. _____
    c. _____
    d. _____

19. List eight indications for CPAP in the neonate.
    a. _____
    b. _____
    c. _____
    d. _____
    e. _____
    f. _____
    g. _____
    h. _____

20. List six factors that constitute the physical examination indicators for the use of CPAP.
    a. _____
    b. _____
    c. _____
    d. _____
    e. _____
    f. _____

21. What are the blood gas values that indicate a need for CPAP?
    _____
    _____

22. List two findings on chest radiograph that may indicate the need for CPAP.
    a. _____
    b. _____

23. List five conditions that are thought to respond to CPAP and which are associated with one or more of the previously listed clinical presentations.
    a. _____
       _____
    b. _____
    c. _____
    d. _____
    e. _____

24. What are the two general approaches used to minimize the use of mechanical ventilation and protect the neonatal respiratory system?
    a. _____
    b. _____

25. What does InSURE stand for?
    _____

26. List two clinical situations where CPAP therapy can be dangerous to an infant.
    a. _____
    b. _____

27. When may infants require intubation and mechanical ventilation rather than CPAP?
    _____
    _____
    _____
    _____

28. List three methods of delivering CPAP to newborns.
    a. _____
    b. _____
    c. _____

29. What are the most critical facts concerning the application of CPAP interfaces?
    _____
    _____
    _____

30. What should CPAP stabilizing equipment be periodically checked for?
    _____
    _____
    _____

31. List the five components that make up a CPAP system.
    a. _____
    b. _____
    c. _____
    d. _____
    e. _____

32. List four problems that improper positioning of the nasopharyngeal (NP) tube can cause.
    a. _____
    b. _____
    c. _____
    d. _____

33. How is pressure regulated in bubble CPAP machines?
    _____
    _____

34. What is the initial pressure setting for CPAP, and how should the CPAP level be adjusted?
    _____
    _____

35. What is considered an adequate level of CPAP?

    _____

    _____

36. List 10 possible complications of CPAP.

    a. _____

    b. _____

    c. _____

    d. _____

    e. _____

    f. _____

    g. _____

    h. _____

    i. _____

    j. _____

37. List four complications that accompany neonatal endotracheal intubation.

    a. _____

    b. _____

    c. _____

    d. _____

38. List four uses of noninvasive positive-pressure ventilation (NIV).

    a. _____

    b. _____

    c. _____

    d. _____

39. Suggest initial intermittent mandatory ventilation settings for neonates.

    _____

    _____

    _____

    _____

40. Describe SiPAP and list the common settings.

    _____

    _____

    _____

41. What are the benefits of bilevel positive airway pressure (BiPAP) and NIV in the pediatric population?

    _____

42. Suggest initial settings for a pediatric patient receiving BiPAP.

    _____

    _____

    _____

43. List four major categories of indications for mechanical ventilation in the neonate.

    a. _____

    _____

    b. _____

    _____

    c. _____

    _____

    d. _____

44. List seven diseases/syndromes that can reduce the lung compliance and/or increase the airway resistance in a neonate.

    a. _____

    b. _____

    c. _____

    d. _____

    e. _____

    f. _____

    g. _____

45. List four diseases/syndromes that impair the cardiovascular function of a neonate.

    a. _____

    b. _____

    c. _____

    d. _____

46. List five indications for mechanical ventilation of pediatric patients.

    a. _____

    b. _____

    c. _____

    d. _____

    e. _____

47. What are the arterial blood gas indicators of respiratory failure in pediatric patients?

    _____

    _____

48. Historically, what is the most common modality used to ventilate infants?

    _____

49. In an infant ventilator, what type of trigger avoids breath stacking and asynchrony?

    _____

50. Discuss the difference between continuous flow and demand flow for spontaneous breaths.

_____

_____

51. What triggering methods are available for neonatal and pediatric patients?

_____

_____

52. What is the preferred triggering method for neonates? Why?

_____

_____

53. What is the major limitation of proximal flow sensors?

_____

54. Describe how peak inspiratory pressure (PIP) can be optimized during manual ventilation.

_____

_____

55. What is the purpose of positive end-expiratory pressure (PEEP)?

_____

56. What are the acceptable initial PEEP settings?

_____

57. When should PEEP be increased?

_____

58. What is meant by the term *flow chop*?

_____

59. (a) Calculate the time constant when $R_{aw}$ = 45 cm/$H_2O$/L/s and $C_L$ = 0.004 L/cm $H_2O$.

_____

_____

(b) What $T_I$ should be set for this time constant?

_____

60. (a) Calculate the time constant when $R_{aw}$ = 30 cm/$H_2O$/L/s and $C_L$ = 0.002 L/cm $H_2O$.

_____

_____

(b) What $T_I$ should be set for this time constant?

_____

61. What can be done to reduce the potential for ventilator-induced hyperinflation in patients with bronchopulmonary dysplasia or meconium aspiration?

_____

_____

62. What is considered an acceptable leak around a cuffless endotracheal tube?

_____

63. Mean airway pressures greater than _____ have been associated with lung injury in neonates.

64. What $P_aO_2$ levels should be maintained in neonates and pediatric patients?

_____

_____

65. What parameter is set to ensure a tidal volume during volume-targeted ventilation?

_____

66. What factors determine $T_I$ when volume ventilation is used?

_____

_____

67. What types of pediatric patients respond well to volume controlled-intermittent mandatory ventilation?

_____

68. What is the recommended $V_T$ values for PSV?

_____

69. What is a cycling problem that can occur during PSV in patients with an ET or tracheostomy tube?

_____

70. Explain how volume assured pressure support (VAPS) works.

_____

_____

_____

71. What advantage does volume support ventilation (VSV) have over PSV in the administration of surfactant replacement therapy to an infant?

_____

_____

_____

72. How are the pressure levels set in APRV for neonatal and pediatric patients?

_____

_____

73. What benefits does spontaneous breathing at the higher pressure level during APRV provide?

_____

_____

74. What parameters does NAVA allow the patient to control?

_____

_____

75. What are the goals of lung-protective therapy in the neonatal and pediatric patients?

_____

_____

_____

76. When should HFV be considered in an infant's clinical course?

_____

_____

_____

77. List three complications of HFV.

a. _____

b. _____

c. _____

78. Explain the physiologic mechanism of gas exchange in HFV.

_____

_____

79. List the preparations that should be completed before a patient is placed on HFV.

_____

_____

_____

80. What is the general goal for all types of HFV?

_____

_____

81. What do preparations of exogenous surfactant typically contain?

_____

_____

82. Describe the dosing procedure for an exogenous surfactant.

_____

_____

_____

_____

_____

83. Name the two types of toxicity that have been reported with the application of inhaled NO.

a. _____

b. _____

## CRITICAL THINKING QUESTIONS

1. A pediatric patient with a 4-mm ET is receiving PSV. The respiratory therapist notes that inspiration seems to exceed 1 second. What is the most likely cause of this problem and how can it be corrected?

_____

_____

2. VSV has what advantage over PSV during surfactant replacement therapy?

_____

_____

3. An infant receiving nasal CPAP is crying, and each time the infant's mouth opens, the CPAP level on the pressure manometer drops significantly. Why is the pressure dropping and what can be done to correct it?

_____

_____

_____

4. What circumstance can reduce the level of support provided in pressure-regulated volume control? What problems can this lead to?

_____

_____

## CASE STUDIES

### Case Study 1

A 29 weeks' gestation, 2-hour-old infant is in the neonatal intensive care unit (ICU) in an oxyhood with an $F_IO_2$ of 0.5. Physical examination reveals intercostal and substernal retractions, a respiratory rate of 68 breaths/min, and a pulse of 145. The arterial blood gas (ABG) values are as follows: pH = 7.21, $P_aCO_2$ = 70 mm Hg, and $P_aO_2$ = 41 mm Hg. Manual ventilation of this patient demonstrates bilateral chest movement and aeration at 25 cm $H_2O$.

1. The most appropriate PIP setting for this patient is

_____.

During mechanical ventilation, the patient's pressure–volume loop changes from that shown in Figure 22.1, *A*, to that shown in Figure 22.1, *B*.

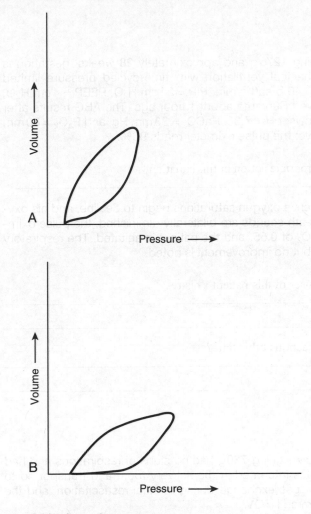

2. What is the most likely cause of this change?

_____

The patient receives Survanta at 2 mL/kg. During this time, the ventilator $F_IO_2$ is increased to 1. Each partial dose is followed by a 30-second period on the ventilator. The pressure–volume loop then takes on the shape shown in Figure 22.2.

3. What is the most likely cause of this change?

_____

## Case Study 2

A newborn male infant weighing 1275 g and approximately 28 weeks' gestation is intubated and receiving mechanical ventilation with time-cycled pressure limited (TCPL) at these settings: rate = 40 breaths/min, PIP = 24 cm $H_2O$, PEEP = 4 cm $H_2O$, $F_iO_2$ = 0.75. The patient received Survanta about 1 hour ago. The ABG results after surfactant therapy were as follows: pH = 7.36, $PaCO_2$ = 38 mm Hg, and $P_aO_2$ = 80 mm Hg. The infant is pink and active; the pulse oximeter reads 96%.

1. What would be the most appropriate action in this situation?

_____

Over the next 2 hours, the patient's oxygen saturations begin to decline, and his oxygen requirements increase. Breath sounds are bilaterally diminished, the pulse oximeter reading is 86% with an $F_iO_2$ of 0.55, and the patient is agitated. The respiratory therapist suctions the patient, but no improvement is noted.

2. Name the two most likely causes of this patient's distress.

_____

_____

3. What is the most appropriate action at this time?

_____

_____

## Case Study 3

A 24 weeks' gestation neonate weighing 730 g had no signs of respirations and had central cyanosis at birth. He was intubated in the delivery room and transported to the neonatal ICU. He had poor gas exchange during manual resuscitation, and the decision was made to place him on HFOV.

1. What should be the setting for the mean airway pressure?

_____

2. The initial frequency setting should be _____ Hertz.

3. How should the initial pressure gradient be set?

_____

## NBRC-STYLE QUESTIONS

1. Which of the following is the best method of ensuring an effective CPAP system?
   a. Use of audible and visual alarm systems
   b. Incorporation of $F_iO_2$ and pressure monitors
   c. Careful monitoring of the patient's work of breathing and oxygenation status
   d. Use of only a mechanical ventilator with continuous flow capability

2. The type of CPAP delivery system that produces vibrations that may have a beneficial effect is which of the following?
   a. Bubble CPAP
   b. Freestanding CPAP device
   c. Mechanical ventilators with CPAP settings
   d. Improvised freestanding CPAP delivery device

3. The safest and most effective method of CPAP delivery to a newborn is with which of the following?
   a. Vapotherm
   b. Hamilton Arabella
   c. Fisher and Paykel bubble CPAP
   d. Improvised freestanding CPAP device

4. In newborns, PEEP is used to accomplish which of the following?
   1. Recruit alveoli
   2. Prevent atelectasis
   3. Decrease the compliance
   4. Establish functional residual capacity
   a. 1 and 3
   b. 1 and 2
   c. 3 and 4
   d. 2 and 4

5. The disease state that prolongs time constants is which of the following?
   a. Acute lung injury
   b. Apnea of prematurity
   c. Bronchopulmonary dysplasia
   d. Respiratory distress syndrome

6. A neonate receiving nasal CPAP of 8 cm $H_2O$ with an $F_IO_2$ of 0.65 has the following ABG values: pH = 7.2, $PaCO_2$ = 69 mm Hg, and $P_aO_2$ = 48 mm Hg. The most appropriate action is which of the following?
   a. Increase the $F_IO_2$ to 0.75
   b. Increase the CPAP to 10 cm $H_2O$
   c. Change to NP CPAP
   d. Intubate and mechanically ventilate with pressure-controlled intermittent mandatory ventilation (PC-IMV)

7. Before an infant is put on PC-IMV, which of the following methods should determine the PIP?
   a. Estimate the PIP for the patient, set the value at a level higher than this, and adjust downward.
   b. Compare chest movement and bilateral aeration with the PIP during manual ventilation.
   c. Estimate the PIP for the patient, set the value at a level lower than this, and adjust upward as needed.
   d. Set the PIP to a safe level, attach the patient to the ventilator, and monitor for improvement in overall appearance and oxygen saturation.

8. Calculate the patient's estimated $V_T$ in PC-IMV when $T_I$ is 0.5 second and flow is 8.75 L/min.
   a. 54 mL
   b. 62 mL
   c. 73 mL
   d. 95 mL

9. $V_T$ is increased during PCV by which of the following?
   a. Increasing PIP
   b. Increasing PEEP
   c. Decreasing flow rate
   d. Increasing $T_I$

10. Which of the following must be monitored during administration of surfactant replacements?
    1. Heart rate
    2. Oxygenation
    3. Temperature
    4. Airway patency
    a. 1, 2, and 4
    b. 2, 3, and 4
    c. 1 and 3
    d. 2 and 4

# 23 Special Techniques Used in Ventilatory Support

## LEARNING OBJECTIVES

*Upon completion of this chapter, the reader will be able to do the following:*

1. Discuss the benefits and disadvantages of airway pressure release ventilation (APRV)
2. Recommend initial settings for initiating APRV in patients with acute respiratory distress syndrome (ARDS).
3. Explain how the controls operate with the Vyaire 3100B High-Frequency Oscillatory Ventilator.
4. Recommend initial ventilator settings for an adult with the 3100B unit.
5. List types of medications that may be used in transitioning from volume-controlled continuous mandatory ventilation (VC-CMV) to high-frequency oscillatory ventilation (HFOV) for an adult.
6. Explain how the chest wiggle factor is influenced by HFOV settings.
7. Name pulmonary pathological conditions in which heliox therapy may be beneficial.
8. Compare the difference between set tidal volume (VT), monitored VT, and actual VT delivery (VTdel) during heliox therapy.
9. Describe how heliox used with a mechanical ventilator may affect pressures and fractional inspired oxygen concentration (FIO2) monitoring and delivery.
10. Explain the procedure for using heliox cylinders with a mechanical ventilator.
11. Name at least four techniques that can help determine the correct placement of the esophageal Edi catheter.
12. Provide examples of how the Edi waveform can be of value in monitoring critically ill patients.
13. Discuss various factors that can cause a low Edi signal and a high Edi signal.
14. Describe the safety backup features and alarms available with Neurally adjusted ventilator assist (NAVA).
15. Calculate an estimated pressure delivery when given the NAVA level, Edi peak, Edi minimum, and positive end-expiratory pressure (PEEP).
16. Explain what parameters (pressure, flow, volume, neural signal, time) are used to deliver a breath during NAVA ventilation.
17. Identify clinical situations in which NAVA should be used.

**KEY TERMS CROSSWORD PUZZLE**

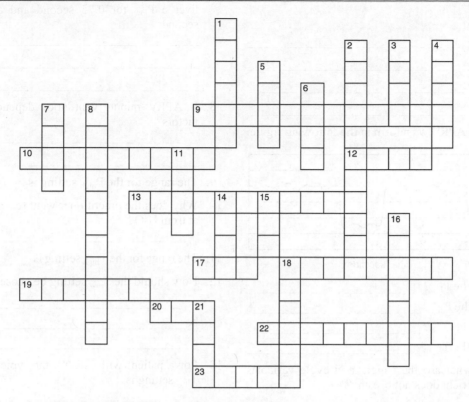

**Across**

9 Region of the lung that receives the most ventilation
10 HFOV control that influences $PaCO_2$
12 Mode of ventilation with two levels of continuous positive airway pressure (CPAP) (abbreviation)
13 Factor observed from the level of the clavicle to the mid-thigh during HFOV (two words)
17 HFOV's equivalent to PEEP (abbreviation)
18 First parameter set in starting HFOV (two words)
19 Helium–oxygen mixture
20 Technique that allows the gas flow to each lung to be controlled separately (abbreviation)
21 Region of the lung receiving the most blood flow
22 A property of helium

**Down**

1 Forward and backward excursion of this device helps determine $V_T$
2 Type of breathing allowed during biphasic CPAP
3 Type of flow waveform produced by HFOV
4 Cycles per minute
5 HFOV is used in the management of this pulmonary problem (abbreviation).
6 HFOV control that directly affects $P_aO_2$ (abbreviation)
7 Heart-lung bypass machine (abbreviation)
8 Brief interval at $P_{low}$ (two words)
11 Type of endotracheal tube (ET) used to accomplish 20 across (abbreviation)
14 Repair of this may cause unilateral lung injury (abbreviation)
15 Applies internal percussion to the lungs (abbreviation)
16 Biphasic CPAP on the Covidien Puritan Bennett 840 (two words)
18 Biphasic CPAP on the SERVO-i (two words)
21 This can be avoided by starting HFOV early in patients with severe ALI/ARDS (abbreviation).

## CHAPTER REVIEW QUESTIONS

1. Define *APRV.*

   _____

   _____

   _____

   _____

2. Refer to the APRV waveform in the following figure.

   a. What is the $P_{low}$? _____

   b. What is the $P_{high}$? _____

   c. What is the $T_{low}$? _____

   d. What is the $T_{high}$? _____

3. In APRV, what are the trigger and cycle variables when the patient does not breathe?

   _____

4. List two other names for APRV that are used in the United States.

   a. _____

   b. _____

5. List four of the physiologic or hemodynamic advantages of APRV compared with other forms of ventilation.

   a. _____

   b. _____

   c. _____

   d. _____

6. List four disadvantages of APRV.

   a. _____

   b. _____

   c. _____

   d. _____

7. Calculate the APRV respiratory rate that would deliver a $P_{low}$ for 0.75 second and a $P_{high}$ for 4.75 seconds.

   _____

   _____

8. In APRV, minute ventilation depends on what two factors?

   _____

   _____

9. The range for the $P_{high}$ setting is _____.

10. Why does the practitioner want to set the $P_{low}$ setting at 0 cm $H_2O$?

    _____

11. The range for the $T_{high}$ setting is _____.

12. How should the $T_{low}$ setting be chosen?

    a. _____

    b. _____

    c. _____

13. For a patient with ARDS, the typical range for the $T_{low}$ setting is

    _____

14. List the three factors that determine ventilation and $PaCO_2$ in APRV.

    a. _____

    b. _____

    c. _____

15. Describe one method of weaning a patient from APRV.

    _____

    _____

    _____

    _____

16. HFOV oscillates the lungs at what rates?

    _____

17. What creates the high-frequency oscillations in the SensorMedics 3100B?

_____

18. What determines $V_T$ during HFOV?

_____

_____

19. What determines the appropriateness of the power setting?

_____

_____

20. Increasing the HFOV frequency does what to patient ventilation? Explain.

_____

21. Reducing the HFOV frequency does what to patient ventilation? Explain.

_____

22. What does the $T_I\%$ represent on the SensorMedics 3100B?

_____

_____

23. How does the bias flow setting influence the patient's $PaCO_2$?

_____

_____

_____

24. List the indications for HFOV in adults.

_____

_____

_____

_____

25. What is the one exclusion criterion for use of the SensorMedics 3100B?

_____

26. List the types of medications that may be used in transitioning from VC-CMV to HFOV in an adult.

_____

_____

27. A patient on HFOV may be checked for a return to conventional ventilation when what two parameters have been reached?

_____

28. Describe the physical characteristics of helium.

    _____

    _____

29. List the pulmonary pathologies that may be treated with heliox therapy.

    _____

    _____

30. Calculate the actual flow reading for an 80:20 heliox mixture with a displayed flow rate of 6 L/min.

    _____

    _____

31. Complete the following table, which compares volumes delivered during heliox therapy provided by critical care ventilators.

| Ventilator | Volume With Heliox |
|---|---|
| CareFusion AVEA | _____ |
| Hamilton Veolar and Hamilton Galileo | _____ |
| Covidien Puritan Bennett 840/980 | _____ |
| Servo-i | _____ |
| Drager Dura-2 | _____ |
| Drager E-4 | _____ |
| Hamilton G-5 | _____ |
| Servo-u | _____ |

32. How is heliox connected to a mechanical ventilator?

    _____

    _____

33. How does the use of heliox with a mechanical ventilator affect $F_1O_2$ monitoring?

    _____

    _____

    _____

    _____

34. How does the use of heliox with a mechanical ventilator affect pressures?

    _____

    _____

35. Name a circumstance in which heliox therapy should not be used.

    _____

    _____

36. Compare synchronous with dyssynchronous ventilation when two ventilators are used for ILV.

_____

_____

_____

_____

_____

37. Define the expiratory inflection point. What is another term used to describe it?

_____

_____

38. What should the mode, rate, and $V_T$ be for performing a less hemodynamically stressful slow-flow inflection maneuver to one lung? To both lungs?

_____

_____

39. How are appropriate levels of PEEP established for each lung during ILV?

_____

_____

_____

40. How is ventilator triggering established during NAVA?

_____

_____

41. List two backup modes set when a patient is being ventilated in the NAVA mode.

a. _____

b. _____

42. List five conditions that would exclude a patient from the use of the NAVA mode.

a. _____

b. _____

c. _____

d. _____

e. _____

## CRITICAL THINKING QUESTIONS

1. What ventilator mode and settings are represented by the following pressure–time graph?

_____

_____

2. After an adult patient is placed on HFOV, a chest radiograph shows the diaphragm in the midclavicular line to be at the level of the sixth posterior rib. Which ventilator parameter, if any, needs to be changed and why?

_____

_____

For Questions 3 through 5, refer to the pressure–volume curve for a slow-flow inflection maneuver displayed in the following figure.

3. Plot the lower inflection point and the upper inflection point for the static pressure–volume loop.

_____

4. PEEP should be set at what level?

_____

5. What $V_T$ should be used to ventilate this patient?

_____

## CASE STUDIES

### Case Study 1

A patient is ventilated with APRV at the following settings: $P_{high}$ = 20 cm $H_2O$, $P_{low}$ = 2 cm $H_2O$, $T_{high}$ = 4 seconds, $T_{low}$ = 1 second, $F_IO_2$ = 0.4. The patient's spontaneous rate is 12 breaths/min. The current arterial blood gas (ABG) values include a $P_aO_2$ of 86 mm hg and a $PaCO_2$ of 68 mm Hg.

1. Calculate the current ventilator rate.

   _____

   _____

2. Which parameter needs to be changed to correct this patient's problem?

3. State the reason for changing that parameter.

   _____

   _____

### Case Study 2

A patient currently is ventilated with APRV at the following settings: $P_{high}$ = 35 cm $H_2O$, $P_{low}$ = 5 cm $H_2O$, $T_{high}$ = 7 seconds, $T_{low}$ = 0.5 second, $F_IO_2$ = 0.3. The patient's spontaneous rate is 14 breaths/min. The current abg values include a $P_aO_2$ of 58 mm Hg and a $PaCO_2$ of 42 mm Hg.

1. Which parameter needs to be changed to correct this patient's problem?

2. State the reason for changing that parameter.

   _____

   _____

3. If changing this parameter does not correct this patient's problem, what other change could be made?

   _____

   _____

### Case Study 3

A male patient, 6 feet 2 inches tall and weighing 81 kg, underwent thoracoabdominal surgical repair of an aortic aneurysm and has been brought to the surgical intensive care unit. He is intubated with a double-lumen ET tube, and two ventilators are ready at the bedside.

1. Which lung will have sustained injury as a result of the surgery? Why?

   _____

   _____

   _____

2. What volume should be used in this patient to perform a single-lung slow inflation maneuver to determine inflection points?

3. If the right lung's lower inflection point is 6 cm $H_2O$ and the left lung's lower inflection point is 18 cm $H_2O$, what is the appropriate PEEP level for each lung?

   _____

   _____

## NBRC-STYLE QUESTIONS

1. The advantages of APRV over other forms of conventional ventilation are mainly the result of which of the following?
   a. Preservation of spontaneous breathing
   b. Reduced risk of ventilator-induced lung injury
   c. Reduced risk of ventilator-associated pneumonia
   d. Reduced need for patient sedation and paralysis

2. Which of the following are the most appropriate APRV settings for an ARDS patient who is receiving VC-CMV at these settings: rate = 12 breaths/min, $V_T$ = 600 mL, $F_IO_2$ = 1, PEEP = 10 cm $H_2O$, peak inspiratory pressure = 32 cm $H_2O$, $P_{plat}$ = 25 cm $H_2O$?
   a. $P_{high}$ = 42 cm $H_2O$, $P_{low}$ = 10 cm $H_2O$, $T_{high}$ = 2 seconds, $T_{low}$ = 2 seconds
   b. $P_{high}$ = 25 cm $H_2O$, $P_{low}$ = 10 cm $H_2O$, $T_{high}$ = 4 seconds, $T_{low}$ = 2 seconds
   c. $P_{high}$ = 25 cm $H_2O$, $P_{low}$ = 0, $T_{high}$ = 4 seconds, $T_{low}$ = 1 second
   d. $P_{high}$ = 15 cm $H_2O$, $P_{low}$ = 0, $T_{high}$ = 6 seconds, $T_{low}$ = 1.5 seconds

3. The parameter that can generally improve oxygenation during APRV is which of the following?
   a. $P_{high}$
   b. $P_{low}$
   c. $T_{high}$
   d. $T_{low}$

4. Calculate the APRV ventilator rate when $T_{high}$ is 12 seconds and $T_{low}$ is 2 seconds.
   a. 4 cycles/min
   b. 6 cycles/min
   c. 9 cycles/min
   d. 12 cycles/min

5. The first parameter set when starting HFOV is which of the following?
   a. $T_I\%$
   b. Frequency
   c. Amplitude
   d. Bias flow

6. A decrease in chest wiggle during HFOV may be caused by which of the following?
   1. Pneumothorax
   2. ET obstruction
   3. Increased $PaCO_2$
   4. Patient improvement
   a. 1 and 2
   b. 2 and 3
   c. 4
   d. 1 and 3

7. An ARDS patient is receiving HFOV at the following settings: $P_{aw}$ = 28 cm $H_2O$, frequency = 6 Hz, bias flow = 30 L/min, $\triangle P$ = 7 (amplitude 60 cm $H_2O$), $T_I\%$ = 33, $F_IO_2$ = 0.8. The patient's $P_aO_2$ on these settings is 75 mm Hg. Which of the following is the most appropriate action in this case?
   a. Increase the $F_IO_2$ to 0.9.
   b. Reduce the control to 5.
   c. Reduce the frequency to 5 Hz.
   d. Increase the $P_{aw}$ to 30 cm $H_2O$.

8. With HFOV, the first step in reducing an adult patient's $PaCO_2$ is which of the following?
   a. Increase the $T_I\%$.
   b. Reduce the frequency.
   c. Increase the amplitude.
   d. Increase the cuff leak.

9. To achieve a flow of 8 L/min for a 70:30 heliox mixture, the oxygen flowmeter should be set at which of the following?
   a. 5 L/min
   b. 8 L/min
   c. 11 L/min
   d. 14 L/min

10. With HFOV, volume delivery from the oscillator is determined by all of the following, except:
    a. $T_I\%$
    b. Oscillator displacement
    c. ET tube size
    d. Patient's ability to trigger the ventilator